Miles To Go Before I Sleep

Letters on hope, death and learning to live

CLAIRE GILBERT

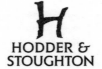

HODDER &
STOUGHTON

First published in Great Britain in 2021 by Hodder & Stoughton
An Hachette UK company

1

A CIP catalogue record for this title is available from the British Library

Hardback ISBN 978 1 529 35972 5
eBook ISBN 978 1 529 35974 9

Typeset in Bembo MT by Hewer Text UK Ltd, Edinburgh
Printed and bound in Great Britain by Clays Ltd, Elcograf S.p.A.

Hodder & Stoughton policy is to use papers that are natural, renewable
and recyclable products and made from wood grown in sustainable
forests. The logging and manufacturing processes are expected to
conform to the environmental regulations of the country of origin.

Hodder & Stoughton Ltd
Carmelite House
50 Victoria Embankment
London EC4Y 0DZ

www.hodderfaith.com

For Seán, who is the true hero of this story

Contents

Prologue

I write, because I'm going to die.

Writing has always been my way of trying to make sense of things, so it was to writing that I turned when I heard I might have cancer. Then, on impulse, I asked a group of family and close friends: Will you read what I write? You don't have to respond, I said. Just be my Dear Readers. Because you love me I will be able to write with complete honesty. I won't have to put on a brave face or edit my words to avoid offence. I won't have to pretend.

I have myeloma, an incurable cancer of the blood. I can't defeat it; I have to live with it. My blood flows through every part of me, bringing me life as well as, now, the promise of death. I will not let cancer be the cause of bitterness growing in me. But until I started writing to people who love me, I didn't know how I was going to make this happen. Now, the unfailing kindness of my Dear Readers meets my visceral need and the words that emerge teach me how to put my cancer to work and how to make it a source of joy. And they are interwoven with equally honest words from the Dear Readers who thankfully ignore my request not to respond. They have supported me more than I can say and still do: they have grown in number and I continue to write to them.

My Dear Readers have given me many gifts. One is the permission to write of my pain even though I struggle with the feeling that I have been let off lightly. I have many material privileges to cushion my experience and I have been consistently humbled by the strength of my fellow cancer sufferers, all of whom seem to carry greater burdens than I. The Dear Readers allow me to acknowledge how hard it nevertheless is: I still reel from the diagnosis and am made sick by the treatment and no amount of privilege protects me from that.

What human being, whoever they are, has not or will not face deep, disconcerting challenges in their lives that send them reeling? It's not just about you, say the Dear Readers, so write about it, because you can. And that is how the private correspondence has come to be published.

This book reproduces the 2019–20 Dear Readers' letters, which take the form of a diary unfolding in real time.* You join me in my stumbling walk of discovery and my attempts to make sense of it all. In among the treatments and horrible side effects, the Dear Readers and I converse about death and life's purpose; turn to nature and horses; turn to Julian of Norwich (I wrote my doctoral thesis on her; now she teaches me); feel profound gratitude for friendship and material comforts; tell jokes; pull on brightly coloured clothes and wear lipstick and pearls to chemotherapy; quote poetry; and then, when we'd been through enough already, face the threat of Covid-19 together.

The walk will at some point come to an end. Mitterand said 'death is an accomplishment',[1] because it is only then that a life makes sense, when the full magnificent picture of it can be seen. But, as I have discovered, there are many miles to go before that final sleep, and the miles we walk actively create meaning and the meaning is beautiful.

Dear Reader, for you are one now, I invite you to walk with me. I place no carapace around my vulnerability. I risk your eyes on my raw physical and emotional self. Walk with me. Don't walk away.

* Individuals are identified by their name initial where appropriate, in both the letters and playlist at the end of the book. Other characters' forenames appear in full and have been changed where it has not been possible to gain their permission for inclusion.

I

Diagnosis

First Letter

Dear Readers

Friday, 18 January

It's twenty hours since Dr Adam told me I have a protein that might be myeloma, a cancer of the blood. What an extraordinary and yet utterly ordinary thing to be told: that you might have a life-threatening condition, that you might die. Because of course I am going to die anyway. The one certainty about being born is that one's life will end. And the shock of its possibility, perhaps sooner than one thought (but one doesn't think, that's the truth of it) is, I am finding, rather liberating. At last: an absolute in my life that puts everything else into perspective. I am breathing the air, loving Seán, connecting with Nutkin, the horse I ride this morning, seeing the sky, adoring the view of the Old Town from my eyrie in our house in Hastings, receiving the mighty view of the sea, enjoying the crunchy tang of an apple, and so on and so on: accepting the present moment and loving it. And I'm not finding myself thinking that I will miss it, nor that I want to hang on to it. It is so precious, and it is itself. It will survive me and that matters more, now.

I was in the pub in Hastings Old Town when the doctor phoned. Sitting enjoying a pint with Seán, just off the London train. Dr Adam said: If you do have it, the treatments aren't too bad. You don't get sick or lose your hair or anything.

But still. Cancer.

I went to the cloakroom and looked straight into my own eyes in the mirror above the sink, and I saw strength enough for this. I shall

– I *shall* – be a good companion for myself on this journey, whatever it entails (and it may entail nothing).

The Damocles' sword of cancer has hung over me and you, my dear siblings, for a long time. It's what our family dies of if the last two generations are anything to go by. I have been silently waiting for one of us to succumb.

And in contemplating the possibility that it might be me, I make the discovery that it is (at the moment, anyway) worse to be the loved one of the ill one, rather than the ill one herself. When it happens to you, you face it. When it happens to one whom you love, it undoes you. Cancer – illness, death – is profoundly social. And that is going to make it much, much harder.

For however ready I might be to face my own death, Seán is determined that I will outlive him. He declaims as much with the voice of God over the dinner table that night. And how can I wish to die before him? His wife died suddenly, in a car crash, too soon.

Sunday, 20 January

Deep tears rising to just below the surface of me. I resolutely think of other things, or repeat *maranatha* (an Aramaic mantra meaning 'Come, Lord') like a talisman. I do not allow myself to investigate 'myeloma' online; the endless imaginings and plannings that will attend knowing the prognosis and treatment should be delayed as long as possible, ideally until after I know for certain that I have it – for, of course, I may not. Today I feel so well, so normal, and Seán really is not well, that it seems indulgent to imagine anything about cancer and dying and death for myself. The deep tears abate.

Dr Adam rang again yesterday to talk about checking his diagnosis. He is a nephrologist: I had gone to him to have my kidneys checked. He needs to hand me over to the oncologists.

I can't do anything about this until tomorrow. Agitation and unhappiness flare up over organising the necessary tests. Death I can face, I think, but endless complicated arrangements for its prologue distress me.

I read *Lucia in London* by E.F. Benson. It happens to be the book I am reading here in Hastings and its frivolity irritates me but then it quickly becomes a comedy so charming and delightful that it brings life back to my life. Benson makes me relish what is, in all its absurd beauty.

I'm trying an imaginative exercise of letting love flow into my blood and around my body, imagining the love washing through my blood and all the cells and proteins in my blood, so if the cancer is there it is being washed in love.

Fr Eamonn speaks at mass about the story of the wedding feast at Cana in relation to what Jesus offers when we are nothing but jars of water: if I am empty of everything and don't have anything left to give, his miraculous grace gives me not just more of the same but a transformed self. Yes. Cana wine. I can try that.

Monday, 21 January

I am scared. Today we travel back to London and I have to start taking action to find out if this blessed protein is cancerous.

I have to tell some close colleagues the situation because I may not be able to keep my countenance and they should know why. But it will be shocking: the fact that nothing is yet confirmed does not stop imaginations firing up.

I can work. I have decided what I am going to say in my lecture on justice in public life. Thank God, thank God for work and the ability to focus.

On my own in the evening, I drink champagne, toasting *l'chaim*. Life. The great teaching in this time for me is to do what, citing Plato, I have advocated for decades: live as though you are going to die today. And that brings life to life like nothing else: vibrant, shouting, dancing, loving life. The champagne is vintage and delicious.

I weep.

Just below the surface there are not only exquisitely painful tears whose origin is deep within me, but also a pumping stress. I can think calmly of only one thing at a time, so that is what I shall do. If I start to multiply my tasks and decisions, I am immediately in distress.

No appointments yet. You tell me this is the hardest time, J, you who have had cancer: when you don't yet know. My way of dealing with it is to let myself imagine the worst (whether that is outright death or ghastly ongoing treatments I'm not sure – the latter I think), but very gently, as though probing a tender wound, a place of great hurt and vulnerability. It hurts but it is life-giving.

Wednesday, 23 January

Today the deep tears and anxiety are right on the surface. I am breathing carefully, focusing on one thing at a time, asking nothing difficult of myself. I am alone so I let the tears fall. And I write this, now, and it calms me.

Despite my mortal fears, I also see, now as I write, the prospect of death as exciting. At last ultimate questions might be answered. At last that of which I have caught glimpses might be in plain sight and not partially, but wholly, what is. I remember Patrick Mayhew's five-year-old granddaughter piping up in her prayer at his memorial service: 'I hope you have lots of adventures in heaven'. I don't know what happens when we die. I don't know if there'll be a 'me' to experience anything. But if this life has taught me anything, it has taught me that love is its final truth, its meaning, as Julian of Norwich puts it. So when the mortal things are put aside and that which has to come to an end does come to an end, what will be left, I believe, is love. And it is magnificent.

You say you will pray for Seán, J. You say that when you had cancer it was far, far harder for your partner than for you. And it's true that if it weren't for Seán and others whom I love and who love me, I would have little hesitation about embracing death. While I certainly do fear and dread illness, I feel I could face it more readily and bravely if I didn't have to worry about its effect on those who love me. But of course the last thing that loved ones want is to be a burden on the sufferer. What a conundrum of human interdependence. As you say, J, our humanity is found in each other. Love is our gift to each other, but it is costly.

I passed an excessively painful stool yesterday, which seemed to be stuck in a muscle in my anal sphincter. The pain was so great that it brought on waves of nausea and I came close to fainting. While it was happening, all I could wish was that it would come to an end.

All I could manage was to breathe and try gently to dislodge the stool. Finally it passed, with no after effect that I could feel. The nausea and faintness went away.

Pain, like love, has to be experienced if it is to be known. That is Julian's vision.

Meanwhile Seán, having gone to hospital for some tests, has been kept in. He is being a completely lovely patient, glad to have the tests he needs to find out what is wrong. His blood is showing an acute inflammatory response but no one knows what to. Not, we think now, an infection. He has absolutely no energy and drenches his bed with night sweats. But he is in good spirits. My potential illness is bracing him, and his illness is in turn making me determined to remain serene throughout the next few weeks and months.

Friday, 8 February

It is disconcerting walking into Guy's Cancer Village (village? really?) for the first time. You have to check in at machines, just like at the airport, except they are so characteristically NHS that I have to laugh, for all my disconcertedness. You touch the screen and it asks you to scan the barcode on your appointment letter. I look at my appointment letter. No barcode. So then I go through a question-and-answer process as if I have forgotten my appointment letter (I haven't!) and the machine recognises me and tells me that my name will come up on the big screen informing me where to go. I look at the big screen; it isn't working. Luckily there are some lovely kind human beings around who help my nervous helplessness. Then I walk past a shop and wonder what a lingerie outlet is doing in the Cancer Village (it's a *building*, not a village) until I see not only bras but also wigs. That really brings it home to me. Bras for mastectomies. Wigs for baldness. And I am here in this place for people with cancer and I am a person who may have cancer.

The consultant, Dr Inas, is kind. Right at the end of our conversation I tell her that my partner is in hospital and I break down in tears. She says, 'Whatever this is, we can treat it.'

Tuesday, 12 February

I return to the Cancer Village for a full body MRI scan, to find out if there is any evidence of myeloma lesions in my bones. Myeloma attacks your bones. (God help me: both my parents' cancers had them gasping with the agony of bone pain.) This time I have a barcode and proudly scan it. The machine doesn't respond. I am late and anxious. A volunteer comes over and explains that the barcodes at the bottom of appointment letters don't work, only the ones at the top. Mine is at the bottom. Silly me. So again, with her help, I circumvent the barcode and type in my details as if I have forgotten my appointment letter (am I going to be marked down as an amnesiac?), but this time the machine doesn't recognise me at all. So the nice lady takes me up in the lift, which features calming birdsong, and delivers me to the right place while I grumble about the inappropriate use of AI.

The message about my claustrophobia has not been conveyed to the radiologist in charge. But the scanner is a doughnut with a big hole for my body to pass through, not the narrow, closed tunnel I had imagined, and I survive without making an ass of myself in front of the beautiful young people attending me.

Monday, 25 February

The haematology department where my bone marrow biopsy is to take place is in the main building of Guy's Hospital and does not exude the determined cheerfulness of the Cancer Village. None of the pastel soft furnishings, big spaces, floor-to-ceiling windows and balconies with plants and views across the river towards Parliament, numerous kind and upbeat volunteers, coffee hubs, soothing birdsong recordings in the lifts and reflexology if you want it. Here we are in standard NHS blue plastic chairs, crowded into a room in the 1960s Southwark Wing, with busy nurses in red shirts (haematology, geddit?) and a lot of waiting. At least there is no underdeveloped AI technology to fail to communicate with: when I arrive and my wrist label is not in the pile with the others a receptionist is there to sort out the stalled printer. I am currently more aware than usual of people's facial accoutrements, as I have just had my eyebrows tattooed (anticipating hair loss despite the doctors' reassurance, but they needed it anyway), but even if I hadn't I think I would have found this young receptionist's mouth and eyes startling. The eyelashes are like the brushes you used to see on Ewbank carpet sweepers – remember the comments on Princess Diana's mascara'd eyelashes when she attended that operating theatre? Are these hygienic? I ask myself – and the lips are blown up and pushed out into the most enormous pout. They look really painful. She herself is childlike, charming and kind, loves the fact that we both have birthdays in October, and I love the fact that she doesn't comment on how many decades there must be between our Octobers, even in her facial expression. Though that would be difficult. *Smiling* looks difficult.

Talking of pain. I am found by a delicate-featured, lithe young boy who takes me into a little room containing a bed on which is spread a pad that looks ominously like something you'd use for incontinence. 'I'm the doctor who's going to do your biopsy. Is that all right?' He is a bit like those sweet, needy waiters you get in vegan restaurants in Brighton. He proudly shows me all his instruments, newly unwrapped and neatly laid out, and I nod admiringly, and then he explains that patients usually only feel pain when the needle is right in the bone and he is removing the 'honey' – the aspirate or proto-blood that's made in the marrow – and the 'honeycomb' – the trefoil or structure of the marrow – of both of which he needs a sample. 'It's a *sucky* kind of pain,' he says, brightly. He is having the effect those needy waiters have, making me want to reassure him rather than the other way around.

Little do I know . . . I lie on the bed on my side. 'Pull your top up a bit further, we don't want to get any blood on it,' again brightly. He is behind me because the biopsy is taken from the back of the hip, but he explains everything that he is doing, taking a kind of chef's pride in it. 'There, now we have a completely sterile area,' surveying my upper backside after he's cleaned it. And in he goes with his anaesthetic needle and then the biopsy needle, the size of which, luckily, I can't see. He is lovely, actually, getting me to talk about my work while the needle bores its way into my bone. Naturally we start talking about Brexit as soon as I mention

Westminster, and I find myself pleading with him not to disengage from politics – 'I'm going to stop voting,' he declares. 'I always did vote but I just don't see the point anymore' – but it's quite hard to develop a reasoned argument about the undermining of democracy and the rise of extremism when you are IN AGONY and I say politely that I have to stop talking and start shouting at the pain, if that's all right? The noise I make is a lot like a birthing mother. It definitely helps. An excruciating pain inside my bone, and a shooting pain down my leg, which feels like really bad sciatica, and which turns out to be a good indication that he is in the right place. '*Sucky* pain'?? He tries to draw out the 'honey'. You're not giving me any samples,' he says, sorrowfully. I am a failure. He has to go in again, and then I am flooding him with the stuff, he exclaims. Then more anaesthetic (which works up to but not in the bone itself, and not on the sciatic nerve, clearly) and in again with a different needle to cut out some of the 'honeycomb'. Even more excruciating. 'In, and I'm just going to turn the needle and – this will hurt' – MORE? – 'and out it comes . . . I'll just take a look at it . . . Oh.' He shows me the sample: a little curled up worm dropped into a jar of solution. 'It's not really long enough.' He needs to obtain a centimetre and this is barely half that. So would we send this sample off and risk it being rejected and my having to come back? 'I'm not coming back,' I say flatly. 'Go in again.' It feels like the bravest thing I've said in my life so far. In he goes again, and the second time produces a lovely sample we both purr over, just like the midwives and the mother do in *Call the Midwife* when the baby's been born. 'You have a very strong cortex,' he says, and I feel rather proud of my obstinate skeleton.

Results on Friday week.

Meanwhile Seán is out of hospital, still exhausted, still undiagnosed.

Friday, 8 March

I have the result.

I do have myeloma, an incurable (as it turns out) cancer of the blood. My approximate prognosis, with scientific understanding, current treatments, my own age and state of health (good), is that I will die of the condition in about ten years. Given the amount of research and development in the field, I may live longer because of ever-improving treatments.

I feel strange. Strangely distant from the diagnosis, as if it is happening, yes, to me, but I am also someone else looking on, rather quizzically. A shock which I am probably reeling from, though I do feel quite steady. It helps being on the train to Hastings because that makes me find strength: surrounded by other people I want to hold myself together; I wonder, were I on my own, would I fall apart? My body is trembling a bit. I can't really think about anything else. The newspaper doesn't arrest my attention. Yes, reeling is probably the word for it. But inwardly I do believe I am strong.

I keep thinking of the positives. In ten years I can do a great deal. It's not such a short time as to paralyse me. Seán is relieved that I will, after all, probably outlive him. So many things I don't have to worry about. I'm unlikely to die alone and incontinent in a home. I have no descendants whose futures I will want to see. I don't have to worry very much about money, providing I can keep working for a while.

Grace, the lovely warm clinical nurse specialist, says I should think of myeloma (and indeed a lot of cancers now) as a chronic condition, not a fatal one. That helps me think about how I respond to treatment choices. I won't be beating this cancer, or fighting it. It isn't a war with a winner and a loser. It's my condition. It's part of me, in my blood, my blood which is my life force, which carries so much that is needed all around my body. I love my blood.

I ask Dr Mary when she breaks the news: What should I tell my loved ones? She suggests telling them that I have a cancer which is incurable, but treatable. So let's think of the treatment as something additional that is necessary to life – like eating and bathing and sleeping. Except for the fucking side effects. I don't want to feel sick. And I do not want to get fat on steroids. I am going to remain beautiful until I die.

Yes I am.

The eyebrows are a good start and dying early helps of course. I mean, cancer could be a death of choice if the pain can be managed:

it isn't a paralysing stroke, your body falls apart quite quickly, not bit by bit, and it isn't sudden and shocking like going under a bus, with no time at all to prepare.

I'm going to imagine my ten years. What will I do with them?

I will ride horses and swim in the sea.
I will wear beautiful clothes and good makeup. I will take care of
my skin and my hair and my feet.
I will reread the books I love. Dickens first. He brought to birth
in me my love and respect for words.
I will listen to music; go to concerts.
I will sing.
I will have piano lessons.
I will write. And write and write.
I will write poetry.
I will contemplate. I will learn to contemplate. I will practise
contemplation.

Monday, 11 March

I hold myself together for my appearance on *Start the Week*. It is the hardest thing in the world to get myself up and out to Broadcasting House. I try to stay focused. But the feeling I always have before going on the radio is that I have absolutely nothing to say, so it's hard not to panic. And of course in addition to those normal, difficult anticipatory feelings, I am also walking through a world that has changed utterly for me. As I pass alongside everyone else, on the Underground, through Oxford Circus station, up Regent Street with All Souls, Langham Place, right in the centre of my eyeline, I feel detached. So much doesn't matter. I'm not worrying about the homeless sleepers in the portico of All Souls; I'm not irritated by the pushy commuters; I'm not troubled by the crowds. I feel a huge compassion like a wave engulfing my fellow humans, all of them. Compassion . . . Love . . . Fondness. The feeling you have when you see someone you love doing something ridiculous but because you know them and their motivations and foibles, you watch fondly and with understanding. It feels like that. Including about myself. Perhaps the word is forgiveness. How ridiculous and lovely we all are, walking so purposefully towards . . . well, death.

We gather in the studio where Kirsty Wark is warm and friendly. I begin to enjoy myself, focusing on the conversation. But then to my horror, in order to establish sound levels, Kirsty asks innocently what we each did at the weekend. I freeze. My diagnosis floods like an emotion through me. But answering 'Getting used to my cancer diagnosis' is not an option, so I bark out 'I read my fellow guests' books', which has the merit of being true. And when we start I do have a contribution to make, and Kirsty is a wonderfully constructive interviewer, helping us feel that what we have to say is worthwhile. I can concentrate.

And the feeling of having successfully contributed to an excellent programme is this: fantastic. It has been so hard to get here; I had so wished we could stay in Hastings and hide but I didn't hide, I kept my word and did my work; and it was good. It was a statement of intent. I started (the week, ha ha) as I mean to go on, living with myeloma.

Tuesday, 12 March

And so it is, then, with the lecture. I spend yesterday and most of today polishing it, reading it aloud, making it as good as I possibly can, which includes knowing when to stop editing; there is a moment to stop, and it is not at the point of perfection, it's at the point of knowing I can't make it any better. Because I have worked so hard on it, I am calm before delivering it. And I think because I *have* to be focused I am the most poised I have ever felt at that lectern in the Lady Chapel of Westminster Abbey. There have never been quite so many distractions which I would hitherto have found impossible to tolerate: my microphone seems to hum in accompaniment to my words, just the other side of the walls the Brexit / anti-Brexit demonstrations are at their loudest because the vote on Mrs May's revised deal is to take place tonight, and as if that weren't enough, my poor chairwoman has a dreadful cough. She keeps it very quiet but she coughs. Continually. I keep refocusing, refocusing. My focusing muscle is getting a great deal of exercise and that is probably no bad thing.

Wednesday, 13 March

Because today, finally, I venture to read the sizeable booklet produced by the charity Myeloma UK. It is well written with excellent, clear content. But oh, how hard it becomes to read. Working my way through the symptoms of the disease is like having a tolling bell of doom sounding in my head. Pain: eighty per cent of us have it, from bone disease. And the memories of my mother's pain from fractured ribs caused by her cancer and my father's terrible cries of pain from his bone cancer are there in my heart, instantly. Fatigue, overwhelming tiredness. How can I work if I have that? Bone disease that means they break, especially the ribcage (my mother again) and hips and fractures in the spine that mean you lose height or even compress the spinal cord, and calcium is released from the damaged bone into the bloodstream; infection; anaemia; hypercalcaemia which causes nausea, vomiting, confusion and constipation; kidney damage; and peripheral neuropathy — numbness and pins and needles in my feet and hands.

Now I am frightened. It is one thing to face the prospect of just ten more years of life in good health: what I could do with that time! But it is quite another to live with symptoms like these. And this evening, in the pub after choir, when one of the members asks me vaguely if I'd had my diagnosis — was it something to do with my eye? he can't remember — and I tell him, stupidly, and he responds in a horribly upbeat way — you'll be fine, I have a friend who's lived with it for years — that does not help one little bit because what does he know???, I become very, very upset. Tonight I cry my eyes out, a storm of tears, sobs that feel like being sick.

And inevitably I start thinking I can feel the beginnings of the symptoms. The MRI scan had shown one possible lesion in my right femur. Can I feel something there? Is it real, lasting, imaginary? And is that tingling in my hands? Numbness? I cancel my horse ride, worrying about fragile bones.

Friday, 15 March

I've gained a little perspective. I feel fine. Dr Mary had showed me my results when she told me my diagnosis: there is no calcification, they are uncertain what the MRI femur lesion means, my kidneys are stable. And I am not tired, nor in any kind of pain. Honestly. And if the treatment is to stop the paraproteins proliferating, surely that will stop the symptoms developing?

Now I have just read some more of the booklet and I'm not sure it helps. The ways in which symptoms are addressed are nearly as bad as the symptoms themselves, and culminate in hot water bottles or ice packs to dull the pain. The most important thing is to avoid the symptoms of myeloma. I will accept the side effects of the drugs, if they keep the disease at bay. But high doses of chemotherapy and stem cell transplants do cause nausea and hair thinning and loss, so why did the doctors tell me I wouldn't be sick and most of all I wouldn't lose my hair?

Oh, this is hard. I will be in a much better position to know what to think about symptoms and side effects after next Friday when I will hear what my treatment is to be. Meanwhile (deep breath) I will STOP this train of thought and turn my attention to something else.

Like returning to the list of things I love and want to do now.

You tell me, P, that I must do away with everything except the core: what I am here for, what God wants for me. Get rid of all the dross. Yes.

Saturday, 16 March

Today I feel great. You are a tonic, L: my oldest, dearest friend to whom I can say anything; you know quite naturally how to be with me. Your company simply makes me feel, not better, because I am not in any obvious way ill, but myself. I'm fit as a fiddle and it is crazy not to enjoy that because of fears of an unknown future. Pilates with Glenda is also so therapeutic: she has us gently but deeply working with the muscles throughout our bodies, feeling our way to the ones right in our middles, so that by the time we have finished I am in touch with all of me, and I have awoken my sense of feeling.

I have never before really thought about the connection between 'touch' and 'feel'. Glenda says affirmations don't work (they make me cringe anyway) because they are just words. The question is: What are you feeling? Awaken your imagination to feel your body on the inside. Imagine how it would feel if you were perfectly well. I do so and I do feel perfectly well, and in balance.

And then a pedicure with Elinor, who does a gorgeous foot and lower leg massage, and then a facial. It turns out I can no longer have ultrasound treatment for my face with my diagnosis. Rather than being upset I am pleased there will be no noisy machinery, and my facial is mostly massage with delicious smelling oils. 'Yoga for the face,' Elinor calls it, appropriately. It is marvellous.

This morning I meditate, slowly and clumsily retuning to God, and feeling a great settling in my heart as I remember a verse from the Bible that has long been important to me: 'Seek ye first the kingdom of God, and his righteousness; and all these things shall be added unto you' (Matthew 6:33, KJV). On God I settle my eye; the service to humanity will follow it; the physicians will take care of my body. I ask God to help me put God first.

I have always found God undeniable, but I have found the sentence 'I believe in God' meaningless. I have thought, arrogantly, that God is so around and within me that the 'I believe' sentence is unnecessary. Now I see it is an aspiration. For I am not accustomed to asking God for help, to thinking of God as my guide, aid, support, lover, friend, etc. So while I may have never denied God, I think I have for all these years possibly been denying myself the greatest love I could have had. 'Lord, I believe, help thou my unbelief,' I cry, with Augustine.

I will practise feeling well. Running my attention through my body, feeling each part internally, imagining its wellness, feeling its wellness. Imagining the blood with its over-excited paraprotein production, loving it, soothing it, breathing through it. Look, blood: I have oxygen, calm down, fear not, all is well, no need to create paraproteins for the future, you're storing up what is not needed and it's beginning to hurt you, so fear not, fear not, accept the great gift of life and health and service of the body now.

I am like a house whose front has been blown away, like those houses in the Blitz or a dolls house: open for my insides to be seen;

my beautiful and intimate insides. Open to God; to people's devastating kindness; to their sweet and dreadful clumsy trampling on my delicate floors: Ooh you'll be in pain, you poor thing; but then: Oh my dear, I am here for you; you are loved.

Things not to say to people who have been diagnosed with terminal cancer that might not kill them for a very long time: 'You must be really frightened of what's going to happen.' 'Do you wake up in the night panicking? No? Feeling really sad, then?' 'You'll be absolutely fine.' 'It'll be a breeze.' 'We'll fight this.' 'My [name a relative] died of cancer.' 'I feel your pain.'

I shall try to take these offerings as due reward for all the times I have myself made crass and insensitive comments, or asked questions thoughtlessly in the past, of those on whose side I now am.

Wednesday, 20 March

I was a great advocate of palliative care, not just as 'end of life' care but as the way health care might be offered at any time. After all, I would argue breezily, we're all going to die, so it makes sense to think of health care as always palliative. And shouldn't all health care be directed towards living a happy, flourishing, healthy life? Not just saving life for its own sake, regardless of its quality, which is the governing notion of acute care. But now that I am firmly in the palliative care bracket myself, I can see that there really is a difference. I wasn't wrong to argue that all care is palliative, but the notion of acute care, offered to people who are not named as dying, is in tune with the general will to life that gets us born in the first place, feeds our self-preservation instincts, and feeds that in us which is constantly seeking to learn and grow and develop. It is the will to life in nature generally which gives it the necessary force and energy to evolve against the counter force of entropy.

The conundrum for people in my position is that the very force we need to stay energised and optimistic is the same force that will consistently destroy our peace of mind. Only if I give in to the destructive force of the cancer can I have peace of mind, not if I try and fight it, because I *will* lose. I am going to die, probably of myeloma, so my hopes will be ultimately dashed, even if treatment gives me more years. That is the cruelty of cancer: like a cat playing with a mouse, it raises my hopes only to drop them to the ground again. And it always succeeds in raising my hopes because I want my hopes to be raised; I can't help it. That will to live is what brought me into being.

Hmm. 'Hope' is different from 'optimism', isn't it? Hope remains when there is no reason for optimism at all, resides in me, holding me right now as I countenance my future dying, and it isn't the same as the deluded belief that I will live for ever.

Let me try and stay with calming, quietly enlivening hope, and let go of distressing optimism. And, while I'm at it, pessimism.

Friday, 22 March

Back to the Cancer Village to hear my sentence, following my conviction on 8 March. What a wonderful company I have found myself in: Dr Matthew the consultant and Grace the clinical nurse specialist spend a good two hours with Seán and me, talking over my myeloma diagnosis and the options available. I don't have symptoms (the vague ones I've felt are not sufficient or serious enough to count, it seems) but I do have biomarkers and I should have treatment. That is, the levels of kappa light chains and paraproteins, as they are called (I have both), in my blood are significant. Having been thoroughly frightened by reading about the symptoms of myeloma, I am more than ready to agree. Treatment for me means outwitting (Seán's appropriate verb) the cells that are producing the paraproteins and light chains and hence any symptoms they would cause. If I don't want fatigue and bone pain and bone crumbling and calcification, I need treatment.

I am offered a place on a clinical trial called, for some reason, Cardamon. Four cycles of a new chemotherapy called Carfilzomib; then randomly allocated (to avoid bias) either to a stem cell transplant (the gold standard of treatment) or another four cycles of Carfilzomib. It's thought that the Carfilzomib could replace the transplant, which involves THREE WEEKS in hospital, several months of recovery and I will lose all my hair. I don't lose my hair or even, apparently, feel that sick on Carfilzomib. Being in the trial gives me a chance of avoiding the stem cell transplant. That, to me, at the moment, is the best thing about it.

After all of that, there's another eighteen cycles – EIGHTEEN FOUR-WEEK CYCLES – of maintenance Carfilzomib.

Oh.

I am to become someone for whom strong drugs will be a big part of my life. I who have disdained aspirin. I have a new normality facing me.

Fuck.

But. This is interesting medicine and being part of a clinical trial means I get to contribute. I'm not just a passive recipient but part of the action. This is something else to be interested in, contribute to, learn from, speak and write about. I have written about the ethics of medical research on humans, the theory: now I can write about it from experience, from the inside. And I really like the people I am among, not just the consultants I've met and nurse Grace, but also the patients. They are mostly younger Caribbean men, in whom myeloma is most commonly found. I emerge from the lavatory at the clinic to a great burst of laughter from a family group sitting nearby (not at me, they were just having a jolly time, or making a jolly time). I'm part of that now. And Seán and I are energised, not exhausted, by being in the Village. That's strange, isn't it? I am starting a fascinating new phase of my life, if I can only make it properly part of my life, not a nasty add-on. It can't just be an add-on to my old life because I reckon, for this year anyway, it's going to take up about a third of my time. So I had better embrace it.

Shit.

I am to be a different person. I hope you, my friends, can embrace that newness with me and see how much I want it to be good and true and right and of service. And also funny, and dark and unknown.

Saturday, 23 March

Pilates today is, as ever, deeply healing as I attend quietly to my core muscles, dropping my attention down from my headspace to my wonderful, miraculous body. It is very strong. I can keep my muscles fit, but I have to allow the doctors to attend to my hidden body, my cells, my bone marrow, my light chains. I can't do anything about those. I can only receive and embrace what I am being offered, by people who want me to live, and live well. I find it amazing that they should care about me. It's so particular, almost embarrassing.

But I need also to attend to the thing that only I can attend to, that no doctor or anyone else can, which is my relationship with God. 'Seek ye first the kingdom of God, and his righteousness; and all these things shall be added unto you.' That is my first concern, regardless of what happens to my body. Unlike my job, it doesn't need me to perform in front of others, or be a strong leader or teacher or writer. I need to attend to this first.

Then, when I know what the treatment will involve, I need to attend to my role at Westminster Abbey. I have so much support there, I hope I can do enough to ensure the Institute and its people don't suffer. I'm sure it will be all right – it isn't down to me alone, so it must be all right.

Sunday, 24 March

We read through the information sheet for the clinical trial. Its clarity is exemplary but that means I understand better just how tough it's going to be. Chemotherapy is given over two days each week for three weeks, then one week off. Four times. With numerous possible nasty side effects. Stem cell harvesting (we all have this) requires ghastly growth hormone and other stem cell creation encouragement drugs including more chemotherapy, then a day connected to a machine that removes my stem cells. More nasty side effects. Then randomisation. The stem cell transplant, if I have it, is horrific, a massive dose of chemotherapy that kills lots more of me than just my bone marrow, before my transplanted stem cells bring me back to life; then weeks in hospital and months recovering. The following eighteen months of maintenance chemotherapy might not involve hair loss but I am to expect mood swings and insomnia.

The next two-and-a-half years involve a journey from which I will not, to state the bleeding obvious, emerge unchanged.

Seán suggests a lovely thing to me: that in as much as my cancer is like my mother's (she died when I was twelve; Seán's mother also died when he was twelve, also of cancer), I can think of my going through this ordeal of treatment for her; it is what I would have wanted for her, and she for me, and I can do it. It is in some way redemptive.

Also this thought helps: Socrates liked the idea of losing his body at death because he thought it an encumbrance to pure thought, but he was wrong. My body is as much part of my working out of things as my mind and spirit are; and frankly quantum physics undermines any notion that the three are separate in the first place. Which means that the invasive — really, thoroughly, intensively, painfully, uncomfortably, uglifyingly, nauseatingly, invasive — treatments I am going to have can be thought of by analogy as being struck by a new idea, or having one's mind changed, or deepening one's faith. They will be affordances in my niche, they will be an achievement.

Monday, 25 March

I feel anxious because I want to be in the trial and might not qualify: only six places left! Hurry, hurry! How sweet and ridiculous.

Wednesday, 27 March

From Julian of Norwich:

> See, I am God. See, I am in all thing. See, I do all thing. See, I never lift my hands off my works, nor never shall without end. See, I lead all thing to the end that I ordain it to, from without beginning, by the same might, wisdom and love that I made it with; how should any thing be amiss?

I can only write for myself, not for others who are brought to trial. There will be strength for what is to come. In what is to come there will be great love and goodness, as well as pain and ugliness, but the love is only found in the pain, not despite it, and only by going through it can that be known, and the feeling that God never lifts his hands from his works is only discovered in the middle of those works. Never theoretically.

I read this from Julian: 'The place that Jesu taketh in our soul he shall never remove without end, as to my sight, for in us is his homeliest home and his endless dwelling.' And this morning, meditating, I feel the mantra rather than just recite it, feel the indwelling of God in my breastbone, in the same place where anxiety always grips me just before I have a hot flush, and my soul glows there, and I am at peace.

Just as well. Today I have another marathon session at Guy's, meeting Dr Matthew again and Sarah the clinical trials practitioner who can also take blood, in the grey haematology department where I had my biopsy. I thought I was just popping in to consent to the trial, but there are heaps more questions I find I have to address, including getting rather lost in the scientific detail of the genetic markers it turns out I have for the disease (these are NOT, dear siblings, germline inheritable ones). The disease is so heterogeneous it is impossible for the clinicians to say how I might do or what my prognosis is. Dr Matthew thinks that myeloma is really a dozen different diseases without, yet, the categories to separate it out. Future treatments will be much more personally calibrated, but that can only happen on the basis of big data sets, hence trials like the one I hope I'm going to join.

I may not, because even though I have now consented I have a raft of further tests to pass to ensure I qualify, including more scans – will I be claustrophobic in the scanner at St Thomas', which has a smaller hole than the one in the Cancer Village at Guy's? – and, oh my stars, another bone marrow biopsy. As I leave, I glimpse the beautiful young doctor who had done what now turns out to be only my first biopsy. Not like a needy vegan waiter anymore: now he looks sinister. Sarah takes some blood from me, and rather sweetly tells me that she has been taught how to take blood, but she doesn't do it very often and isn't skilled like the phlebotomists who do it all day. Two slightly bruised arms later, I am inclined to agree. But she is lovely, and I like her, even when she brandishes an ENORMOUS plastic container in which I will have to deposit twenty-four hours' worth of urine at some point. Ugh.

*   *   *

Darling A, thank you for sending me the poem you wrote when we were girls of slender means sharing a house in Oxford:

> Claire, wearing red and laughing,
>   Coming home early, making the tea and talking;
> · The house, surprised from its afternoon sleep in the sun
> Starts alive, and someone passing pauses, unaware
> They've been touched by Claire.[1]

Friday, 29 March

A wonderful ride through the woods and gentle hills of East Sussex. The sun shines and everywhere buds are bursting. The deep quiet of the countryside. The gentle clop of the horses and a shout of laughter or quiet chat or silence in our group. The call of life irresistible. I love it.

H, your bracing companionship is a tonic to my raw psyche. Your belief in me feeds my strength and I am profoundly grateful. You understand me when I say that I am quite excited by the prospect of the year's dreadful challenge. But by the evening, at a private view in an art gallery, I am worn out by other people, and when I wake in the night, I am lonely and wretched.

Seán has said that 'Seek ye first the kingdom of God' means, this year, for me, looking after me. And he's right. But I do find it very, very odd.

Second Letter

Dear Readers

Tuesday, 2 April

Dr Adam, the kidney doctor who found the cancerous paraproteins, sees me for perhaps the last time as I am handed over to my deliverers in the Cancer Village. He wishes me luck. He is the embodiment of humanity and I want to throw my arms around him, only I think I will crush him if I do. Like Dr Matthew, he is small and slight, and carries an air of vulnerability, and a lovely honesty in his speech. I feel better just being with these people. Though there's a lack of awareness of female physiognomy: everyone is given a narrow little tube at reception at the kidney clinic, for a urine sample. I gain enormous smiles of gratitude as I pass along the queue of women at the lavatories handing them plastic cups to assist collection. Peeing into a tube, honestly!

Wednesday, 3 April

I stand still in fear but the Earth keeps turning towards the day when my treatment will start. Day and night, turning, turning, inexorable and pitiless. But (I tell myself gently) the turning will continue once the treatment starts and the days will pass and take me through and eventually away from it. The shortest, darkest day in the year presages longer, lighter ones. The turning is a curse and a blessing, but most of all it is inevitable so I will ride it. I will ride the tigers:

> I am in the jungle. All around me, hidden by the trees and plants, tigers prowl. I am afraid.

I am in the jungle. All around me, hidden by the trees and plants, tigers prowl. But I am in a cage and I feel safe.

I am in the jungle. Now the tigers are in the cage. I wander freely among the trees and plants.

I am in the jungle. There is no cage. I ride the tigers.[2]

Julian of Norwich enters my meditation. I welcome her, allow her to be my teacher. At the beginning of her life she asked for wounds: to experience the pain of Christ's passion and to come so close to death herself that she and everyone around her would believe that she was definitely going to die, in order to transform herself into a better lover of God. Passing through darkness is necessary for transformation, if transformation is what one wants. And I do want. Is this a kind of extreme sport for the soul?

'Wound' and 'wonder' are etymologically linked. Julian continually wonders at her visions and this is what transforms her: she is utterly open to them, like an exposed and vulnerable wound. Her first vision is of the blood flowing from the crown of thorns on Christ's head and of Mary as a young girl at the time of the annunciation. Mary accepts the commission to conceive the human body of God in her own flesh and bring it to birth. Birth is a bloody business itself, wounding the mother. And the Christ she bears becomes wounded, broken and bloody.

I am wounded. Can I think of the cancer as Christ being born in me? The contrary thought pleases me.

Yet another visit to a different part of Guy's, the Cardiothoracic Clinic, for an echocardiogram, because my heart has to be pumping properly if I am to be eligible for the Cardamon trial. Sarah comes down to see me before I go in, joined by two of her colleagues. They cluster around me in the somewhat crowded waiting room full of people in various stages of decrepitude from the very fit to the nearly dead, all there to have their hearts tested, and discuss when I might produce my twenty-four hours of urine sample, another test for Cardamon, with Sarah determinedly handing over the enormous plastic container for the purpose. It looks like something in which you'd keep extra petrol for your car. I would bring it in when I came for my second bone marrow biopsy. I raise the question of having gas and air for the biopsy. Sarah tells me that 'they' — the people who do the biopsies — don't like giving gas and air because it's an additional procedure and increases risk overall. They are only going to take aspirate (that's the liquid proto-blood) not trefoil (the bony honey-comb structure in which it's made) so that would be all right, wouldn't it, she says brightly? No, it wouldn't, I say, realising my voice is rising to panic pitch, not good for the crowd of heart patients. You can have it if you find you need it, Sarah says. And off they go.

Friday, 5 April

I write to Sarah begging for gas and air. I sound like Uriah Heep. But I am starting to feel a pattern is emerging, of acceding to a request on the basis of partial information and then not being able to pull out when the beans are fully spilled. Dr Matthew told me I could have gas and air and on that understanding I agreed to the second biopsy (not that I had any choice if I wanted to be in the trial). Later it seemed the gas and air were not a given. Right at the start, when Dr Adam told me I might have myeloma, he reassured me it was treatable with chemotherapy that would make me neither nauseous nor lose my hair. When I was diagnosed it turned out that there were indeed treatments but the cancer itself is incurable. And at the next meeting: yes, the chemotherapy is given as an outpatient but it's over two days each week and although I might not lose my hair or be sick, I might, because everyone reacts differently; oh yes, and also I will have to have a stem cell transplant which most certainly will mean I lose my hair, and be in hospital for three weeks, and the only way of hoping to avoid that is by being in the clinical trial which would mean a fifty per cent chance of not having the trans-plant. Though I might have to have the transplant later anyway.

One is led by the nose. I think I would have found it impossibly distressing, and also confusing, to receive all the information right at the beginning, so perhaps it is just as well. But I give my consent, and pin my expectations, on what I'm told. I feel again like a mouse being played with by a pitiless cat. I'm trying to find my serenity and hope elsewhere than in treatment options, because they cannot afford to be dashed too often. But being denied pain relief is all wrong.

Julian writes 'how meekly and sweetly and tenderly our maker loveth us'. In my meditation I try to feel this, opening the pores of my soul to love, and slowly, emerging like the dawn or a blush, or indeed a hot flush, I feel it, as the universe loving me, as the faces of my beloved friends and family loving me, as the sea's magnificence loving me, as the birdsong and the hills and the clean air, breath in my body, loving me, as the clinicians at Guy's caring for me: not in the sense of being favoured over others, but still, like the intimate love of a person. I rarely think of or imagine God as a person. God is the universe but God is also the tiniest movement and this love is intimate, personal.

A difficult conversation with HR. HR are not trying to make things difficult, on the contrary, but the official conversation brings home harsh reality. How many days sick leave would I need to take? I cannot say, but I will have to record them. I hear it as a challenge. How few days off sick can I get away with? If I'm not careful I will revert to my self-imposed image of conscientious worker who never takes a break, making myself try and work every day, proving what exactly? If that dastardly stem cell transplant happens, I won't have any choice. Though I can see myself writing in hospital . . . The thing about my work, as Seán points out, is that it is vocational. I don't really stop thinking about the Institute and its work among public servants in Westminster; there's always something mulching away in the compost of my mind. Suppose I have the most brilliant idea just as I am throwing up after chemotherapy? In fact, that is quite likely, because I will make a metaphor even of vomit, just you wait and see, Dear Readers.

Saturday, 6 April

Our house in Hastings is in chaos as darling Maro is painting all the hallways and doors, to get the work done before my treatment starts. The bedroom right at the top of the house, with its newly painted floor, now feels like a captain's cabin in the stern of a ship, appropriately enough since these houses were built for Wellington's officers. From the front windows they could see the pesky French a long way away on the horizon, heading across the Channel from their Norman shores. I am looking now at a fishing boat put-putting towards the harbour arm, returning to the safety of the Fishermen's Beach: not a threat but a solace.

It is all very well for me that the decorating is happening: the smell of paint will have faded by the time I am likely to find it nauseating. But Seán is unwell now, still unwell, and this is not a good environment for him. His breathing is shallow and laboured; he coughs and it hurts; he wakes in the night lathered in sweat. 'Evolving polymyalgia rheumatica' is the latest verdict. The irony is not lost on us: he suffers vile symptoms with a vague diagnosis that brings no clarity of prognosis, while I have absolutely no symptoms with a diagnosis and a prognosis of fierce, bell-like clarity.

I pray for myself and my prayer is soft, asking for the receptive, porous strength I need in order to receive well all that is to come. I pray for Seán and I am a furious, desperate, importunate supplicant: Make him well, God. MAKE HIM WELL.

Third Letter

Dear Readers

I stand as far out as I can on the harbour arm within which the Fishermen's Beach nestles in Hastings Old Town. It's a bit like the Cobb at Lyme Regis but much less pretty: more like a landing strip for a midget plane than a natural feature, ending in machine-handled, vast Cornish granite boulders. But the sweep of it, the crook of it, is pleasing.

I look at the flat grey-green sea, and I look at the peopled land. I can see both in one gaze. The right side of my vision is a still, glassy eternity of water; the left side is busy with dog walkers, beached fishing boats, tall black net huts, garish fun fair rides, sweet stalls and amusement arcades blaring seventies music and the beeps and flashes of gambling games. Hastings stubbornly remains a kiss-me-quick seaside resort despite Old Town down-from-London gentrifiers (otherwise known as Filth: Failed In London, Try Hastings). On my left, the world of the living; on my right . . . eternity? Death? The sea is so still and cold. Which is my world? Both seem strange to me. The birds fly easily between the two.

Tuesday, 9 April

One of the Institute's Fellows has sent me a card and inscribed this poem:

29

For Claire (cf. Matthew 10:29−31)
One day, we shall behold Him − face to Face
And know His glory, see His love for us
In frail flesh, which has known our disgrace.
And in such scene, all earthly gain be loss,
As He wipes every tear − our pride shall wane
And what is now corruptible, put on
A better house than this − which knows no pain,
Thanks to that victory that He has won.
Yet now, as Alexander looked i' earth
We look, and thus are tempted all to dread;
But if we listen, we shall hear the mirth
Of sparrows, and remember what He said.
There are a thousand promises to keep
And miles to go before you come to sleep.[3]

I blink away the tears that start in response to the rallying call − and the faith − of the Robert Frostian final couplet, as I read Tristan's note: 'Frankly, I say it's an excuse to invent a new cocktail and toast fate'. I heartily agree, and hope the researchers enjoy measuring the quantities of gin in my twenty-four-hour urine sample tomorrow.

Wednesday, 10 April

The quality of life questionnaire I am required to complete terrifies me. 'Do you have difficulty walking?' 'Are you in pain?' On a scale of one to five. My answers are all very positive. For now. But why would you have questions about difficulty walking if that is not what is in store for me? I am realising how much the pre-diagnosis Claire was able to dismiss of difficult life experiences: they happened to other people. Even walking into the Cancer Village for the first time I remember now how I thought it wasn't relevant to me: the shop with the bras and wigs; the different floors for chemotherapy and consultation, the people struggling with sticks and baldness. Now, potentially, it all does.

'How worried are you about death,' asks the questionnaire, 'on a scale of one to five?' I have certainly thought a great deal about death; but this question doesn't go anywhere near what I have been thinking.

I am raw as an open wound, jagged as broken glass, lost, worried and distressed. In addition to mounting anxiety as the date for starting chemotherapy moves ever closer, I think I am grieving for the Institute, my baby which I have to relinquish for a time, without yet feeling ready to trust those in whose hands it will be left.

A demanding conversation has left me emotionally devastated and I'm still recovering. Everyone means well. But I feel blundered upon and I hardly know how to help myself.

In Crowhurst Woods picking our way among the delicate, starry, white wood anemones. As we walk, you tell me, N, you who had chemotherapy for your Hodgkin's lymphoma in your twenties, you tell me the image that helped you then: you were a bear struggling through a storm. The storm beat about you as you took one painful step after another, but in yourself you were strong, like a bear, and the storm would − did − eventually pass.

It has taken all weekend to find some equilibrium again. But dread stalks me: as we leave Sunbeam House in Hastings this morning I note that by the time we return I will have received chemotherapy. We are going to Ortigia in Sicily for a few days before the long months of treatment start. Why, oh why, am I about to start on something that will make me feel ill when I feel so well? I do not feel like someone with a terminal disease. I half expect one of the research team to ring me and tell me that the extra tests of last week have shown no myeloma cells in my blood: another traitorous cat-and-mouse thought. But my situation is so counter to the assumptions I have relied upon until now: you only take medicine if you feel ill, and the medicine makes you feel better. Not anymore.

But this thought does not make me believe, for a moment, that I should not go ahead with the treatment. I do trust Dr Mary and Dr Matthew, and nurse Grace, and Sarah and the rest of the team. And there's a part of me that stands aside and looks at what is happening and is deeply interested in it, almost looking forward to the experience to see how I will respond. Writing helps so much because through it I can examine what is happening; not to make sense of it, not yet, but to give thought to it.

And if nothing else this experience is obliging me to surrender control — or rather the desire to control since I don't actually have control — of my Institute, my work, my body, my plans, and acquiesce. I am surrounded by love, cushioned by it, served by it. There is no malice here.

I find myself saying to Dora, my beloved London cleaner, as she weeps and rails at the unfairness of it: it's not unjust. I am strong, so I can do this. In speaking to her I discover that I do indeed have no feeling of injustice. 'What did I do to deserve this?' is not a question I am asking, and I'm not going to start. Bad things happen to good people (assuming I'm good, which I'm not). They just do.

Wednesday, 17 April

I have to trust, and I do trust, the clinical team looking after my body. They know what they are doing. I keep rearing away, like a nervous horse, from any questioning of my care path. I am like a recent convert who cannot bear to have her new-found faith undermined. I bite the head off people who come at me with their own certainties: use this alternative plant-based approach to cancer healing! Use this exciting new approach to destroying the cancerous cells that doesn't threaten your health as chemotherapy does! Are you sure they are right and you really do have cancer? (That question made me *furious*.) Have you looked at X or talked to Y who has lots of experience: she's had cancer; he's a chemotherapy nurse; and so on, and on and on. But I silence people. Cancer has spawned industrial quantities of opinions and options and experiences, and of course we want to share them, and of course they are (mostly) valid in themselves — they have a place in the canon of things to be said or done about cancer. Cancer is on the move like a voracious beast, devouring more and more of us, and everyone's thoughts and efforts can play their part in responding. But all these thoughts and opinions and individual experiences are hypotheses, as all scientific truth is: suggestions that need to be tested, including the care path that I am on. That is why it's so good to be part of a clinical trial: no one is assuming that what I am being given is absolutely the right care path, so it is under investigation in a rigorous context appropriate to the kind of allopathic medicine it is. Randomised controlled trials have improved cancer care beyond recognition: many of us survive cancer now. Other approaches are less allopathic, less capable of being tested in a randomised controlled trial, but they are still capable of being tested in some way, if only epidemiologically, or through qualitative rather than quantitative research. Everything is a working hypothesis until — and here's the delicious rub — it has been disproved. It will be the mistakes in my treatment that will lead to more learning. We learn by our mistakes (so do machines: that, I gather, is the basis of artificial intelligence). The late, great Karl Popper said that a scientist's work is to seek to disprove his hypotheses. Not prove them. Because once you have a hypothesis you find you are committed to it: it is your best explanation of the facts as you have seen them, so you tend to see it demonstrated everywhere. We see the things we are looking for, not the things we don't know about. The scientist's hard task is to look for what she can't yet see, and disproving her beloved hypothesis is the way to do it.

I am not a scientist; I am a patient. My greatest gift to science is to submit myself to the hypothesis that is being tested, and let the scientists see in what ways it doesn't work, because that is how cancer care will progress. For my part, it is entirely rational to thoroughly believe in what I am being offered, because that is giving it its best chance. We know the power of the doctor–patient relationship, how our trust in our healers affects healing; and we know the power of the placebo effect, greater in many cases than licensed prescribed medicines. So my blinkered enthusiasm, like that of the new convert, is a really good thing. Doubt and scepticism are for the scientists, not for me, not now.

But, oh, how it helps that I find myself in a centre of excellence, cared for by highly intelligent, sensitive, thoughtful people. It makes my belief easy.

I feel as a baby must feel when it leaves the womb. The embracing cocoon of work and busyness and being needed has gone, and I am walking in a great space with one set of obligations only, obligations to which I only have to keep saying: Yes.

Now my stomach churns and I am afraid, but I am still strong, like N's bear.

Much, much more importantly, Seán is better. He has energy, and liveliness. Our walk in the anemone-carpeted woods at Crowhurst is evidence of his growing strength. He still coughs, but not so much, he still isn't running marathons, but he's flexible again. My beloved. Thank you.

Fourth Letter

Dear Readers

In Ortigia

Strawberries the size of lemons; lemons the size of pineapples. Strolling without purpose around the old city we come upon sixth-century Jewish ritual baths, discovered in the 1980s in the Guidecca. Deep underground, fed by a natural spring. The water of the *mikveh* (baths) must come from natural sources, not pass through human hands, and the word *mikveh* is connected to *nekaveh*, 'hope':

> Lord, you are the hope (*nekaveh*) of Israel;
>   all who forsake you will be put to shame.
> Those who turn away from you will be written in the dust
>   because they have forsaken the Lord,
>   the spring of living water (*mikveh*). (Jeremiah 17:13)

I relish the connection of living water with hope. Hope doesn't look for happy endings; it is there even when the stories are of unjustifiable and unrelieved horror, like slavery or Auschwitz.

However ghastly having cancer is and however poisonous its treatment, no one – no one – intends me harm. That is quite different from others' suffering at the hands of deliberate or even unintended cruelty. But it has struck me how much of what I am being put through would, in the hands of a hostile other, be classed as torture. The same could be said of course about going to the gym.

Thursday, 25 April

When I skiied, at the end of each day I discovered that my feet ached not only because I had been on them all day, but also because I was habitually pulling them up and away, shrinking from the mountain in an instinctive act of fear. I feel something like that in my psyche now, shrinking away from the truth of my cancer diagnosis, and am trying gently to relax my flinching fear, to walk quietly and slowly towards my psychological pain, and sit with it: this is what St Ignatius teaches when he guides you to feel your way to your place of desolation. You don't try to deal with it or be rid of it. You quietly sit with it, as you might sit with a dear friend who is in great pain which you cannot take away, but you are not going to walk away from them either, so you sit with them.

I have my chemotherapy pep talk, and yet more blood tests, in preparation for the start of treatment next Thursday. I really do believe it will start then, though the PET/CT and PET/MRI scans next Tuesday could in theory still disqualify me from the Cardamon trial.

The pep talk and accompanying literature present more shocks. What a heap of pills I will have to take in addition to the chemotherapy intravenous infusions. And, somehow devastating, my 'week off' chemotherapy every fourth week still requires a visit to the clinic so my hopes for ten days or so away from the Cancer Village are dashed. The regime is astonishing for someone who never swallows a pill. My new cosmos is studded with pills and infusions.

I will be monitored throughout to see if my paraprotein and kappa light chains reduce. It is these which are raised and will cause damage if left to themselves. The monitoring is done through blood tests, monthly twenty-four-hour urine collection (bugger) and a BONE MARROW BIOPSY at the end of the four cycles.

Poor Dr Mary, renamed Dr Cassandra in my mind, who had given me my diagnosis, now has to go through all the possible benefits and the side effects of all the drugs. She has first to explain to me that my treatment will not cure me, but it should improve my survival and control my symptoms. So that is the expected benefit. Then the risks – a barrage of muffled boffs to my psyche as each possible side effect is read out: extreme tiredness; risk of infection; nausea; vomiting; hair loss; sore mouth and ulcers; anaemia; blood clots; leakage around the vein (during infusion if the chemo gets into your tissue and damages it); impaired heart function; impaired kidney function; change in sense of taste; rashes; ringing in the ears; bruising or bleeding; numbness or tingling in the hands and feet; allergic reactions; fluid retention (swollen face and ankles, ugh); irritation of stomach lining and digestion; diarrhoea; sleeplessness; unstable blood sugar; constipation; flu-like symptoms; nail changes. If I haven't had the menopause it will bring it on; if I am pregnant the foetus will be damaged. Dr Mary also writes in specially: 'rare side effect of death on the treatment due to infection'.

I try to get Dr Mary to quantify some of these side effects but she won't be drawn, because the responses to treatment in myeloma are so heterogenous. The shocks are only muffled boffs: you might have them, you might not.

Dr Mary tells me we are having this conversation 'for medico-legal reasons', which makes me laugh and, later, ponder the meaning of consent. In medical ethics and law consent, to be valid, has to be (1) adequately informed, (2) given without coercion, and (3) by a competent person. But my experience of receiving the 'adequate information' when I am still getting used to the idea of having cancer at all makes a nonsense of the legal and ethical requirement. I am not competent, I am incapable of really processing the information I am receiving, so I am not adequately informed because I'm not taking it in; and I certainly feel coerced, not by any person, but by my situation: I have cancer so how can I say 'no' to the treatment? How can my conversation with Dr Mary be classed as consent, however many forms I sign? I say to Dr Mary and afterwards to Grace that what really matters is that (1) you, the clinician, are trustworthy, and (2) I trust you.

The most important thing is not to be complacent about infection, says Dr Mary. Because my immune system is compromised infection could kill me. Grace gives me a thermometer: if my temperature goes above 37.5 degrees I have to phone the helpline and go to hospital and have antibiotics within four hours. But avoiding infection isn't as hard as one might think. I can travel, just not on public transport when it's packed. I have to stay away from people who are unwell. The most likely cause of infection is myself so I have to keep myself clean. Very clean, especially my hands and the inside of my mouth.

I have to eat food from reputable manufacturers and nothing that's past its use by date, and if I have a hamburger I have to tell the person serving that I'm on chemotherapy and please would they cook me a fresh one, not give me one that's been kept warm and waiting for any length of time. This immediately makes me want to go and have one.

There is only one food I have to avoid. I love this. It's green tea.

I have to drink three litres of water a day. That's about six pints. How, exactly, or rather, when? And will I ever leave the house again, since a permanently proximate lavatory will be essential?

Of course if I'm randomised to stem cell transplant then a whole new level of side effects is in prospect, but I can't quite bring myself to read that section of the booklet yet. Partly because I might not have to have the transplant, at least not in this first line of treatment.

I just looked. Oh Lord.

One piece of advice in the booklet I really register is about the difficulty of communicating. I tell myself over and over again that no one wishes me anything other than good things, so even if I find what they say upsetting or irritating or downright tactless, I try hard not to react. I remind myself of all the tactless things I have said in the past to people with cancer. Because more than anything, I need you, Dear Readers, and I don't want you to suppress what you want to say to me when we meet or in response to what you read. And you have written beautiful things to me. Silence is also very restful so please continue to know that you don't have to write.

I would love to hear any jokes, the ones that make you laugh. Also your book recommendations, and poems and prayers that move you.

Sunday, 28 April

In her second revelation Julian of Norwich sees the horrifically disfigured face of Christ on the cross. It is vile, quite unlike his 'fair face' during his lifetime, the most beautiful face of all humanity. And then she writes of being taken in her imagination under the 'broad water' to the sea bed. I am facing changes that I fear will disfigure me; I am about to enter unfamiliar worlds. What will I look like? How will I breathe?

I write down the full drug regime and the potential side effects to help me gain an oversight and some control of what is to happen to me, so that I can prepare myself as best I can to ameliorate it all and keep smiling and sane. But in fact I come away from doing so feeling completely overwhelmed and panicked. Control is the last thing I feel. Vulnerable, exposed and helpless is what I feel. Think about what you can control, I decide, trying to take myself in hand, trying not to give in to the panic. I start to write a diary list of what is to happen on chemotherapy days, thinking about adding in treats, thinking about the book or podcast I will bring to read or listen to while the infusion is happening, thinking about how to avoid infection, where I will buy face masks (but you try finding those kinds of face masks online: all that comes up are the sort that you plaster on your face for beauty, and adding in the word 'protecting' only turned up facials that offer protection against the weather . . . what *is* the technical term for these blessed things?), where around Guy's I will go for long walks on 'dex days' – the day on which I take a massive dose of steroids – to tire myself out, how I will make sure I drink three litres of water a day; I even start thinking about what I will do in hospital for three weeks if I have to be isolated for the stem cell transplant . . . and it is all too much. It is like being rushed off to a holiday when you have had no time to pack properly. The treatment is about to start; I am about to enter an utterly new and unfamiliar world, like Julian's 'broad water' in which I don't even know if I will be able to breathe, and I am completely unprepared. I hate being unprepared.

Seán takes me in his arms as I weep.

It is only long, quiet, tuning-in contemplative prayer that brings some measure of peace to my soul. 'Peace I leave with you; my peace I give you. I do not give to you as the world gives' (John 14:27). Peace will not come from external control because there is only so much I can control. I can only hope to make friends with the cancer and all it entails, respond accordingly, and find my peace deep within myself and deep within all that I encounter: God in all. And, oh, how this becomes the most important thing now. I think I will see if I can meditate rather than read while the Carfilzomib infusion is being given. A challenge to find God in healing poison.

The Julian passage reminds me of the poem 'Breathing Underwater'. Now I reread it, and 'the sea' becomes my cancer. For our family, cancer has always been a neighbour.

I built my house by the sea.
Not on the sands mind you;
Not on the shifting sand.
And I built it of rock.
A strong house
By a strong sea.
And we got well acquainted, the sea and I.
Good neighbours,
Not that we spoke much.
We met in silences,
Respectful, keeping our distance
But looking our thoughts across the fence of sand.
Always the fence of sand our barrier,
Always the sand between.
And then one day
(and I still don't know how it happened)
The sea came.
Without warning.
Without welcome even.
Not sudden and swift, but a shifting across the sand, like wine,
Less like the flow of water than the flow of blood,
Slow but flowing, like an open wound.
And I thought of flight, and I thought of drowning, and I
    thought of death.
But while I thought the sea crept higher till it reached my door.
And I knew that there was neither flight nor death nor
    drowning.
That when the sea comes calling you stop being good
    neighbours,

Well acquainted, friendly from a distance neighbours.
And you give your house for a coral castle
And you learn to breathe underwater.[4]

Tuesday, 30 April

To St Thomas' for the two scans, having fasted for six hours: breakfast was a long time ago and unwelcome at 3.30am. I am filled with radioactive dye and sit, gently glowing, with others in the 'hot' waiting area as the dye spreads around our bodies. My claustrophobia does not rise in me for the PET/CT scan in the biggish doughnut. But the PET/MRI scanner's hole I am slotted into is much smaller and it is hard, very hard. When I am first slid in I make the mistake of opening my eyes and seeing how very close above me – a matter of inches – the ceiling is. I shout and John the radiologist immediately slides me out again and removes the heavy armour that is laid upon me to help me keep still (in other contexts this would be a method of torture). His immediate response has the effect of calming me: knowing that I can be brought out straightaway means I am less panicky about being in, and I say I think I can cope. I keep my eyes firmly closed throughout and say the rosary, picturing each of my fingers for the Hail Marys, my whole body for the Our Father, imagining all the time that I am in a spacious room with a really high ceiling. The machine is noisy, much noisier than the Guy's scanner, bangs and hums that go right through your body, ear-splitting drilling noises, every now and then an instruction to breathe in, breathe out, and hold your breath, for quite a long time, fifteen seconds, John has warned . . . it is an endurance test and I am absolutely at the end of my tether by the time it has finished. But I have managed it, and so contributed to the development of the science of scanning, because now researchers can compare the results from both machines, and will do so again when the scans are repeated after my four cycles of Carfilzomib. Four months to recover. I do hope the research concludes that the CT scanner is perfectly adequate, but I fear this new funky MRI machine will be the preferred diagnostic tool.

Wednesday, 1 May

Oh, Dear Readers, it is now only one day before my treatment starts. All this preparation, all these tests, all these words, all these powerful emotions and thoughts, your endless kind receiving. Wish me well!

II

First Part of the Treatment

Fifth Letter

Dear Readers

Thursday, 2 May

A huge gentle wave of your wonderful messages of support is bearing me up; it carries me to the beach of my treatment with uttermost tenderness and lands me with care.

Last night, the night before my treatment starts, walking back from the station after choir, I felt such a surge of strength and power through my body and soul. I didn't feel invulnerable, I just felt strong.

This morning I read Julian's third revelation of God in a point: 'by which sight I saw that he is in all thing'. Nothing is done by 'happe ne by aventure', and the greatest deed is not greater than the littlest deed, for God does all things. This, she says, was a showing of love.

So today I take this on trust, that God is in all thing, and try not to argue or think of the millions of horrific evil things that happen every day to innocent people and creatures. Today I trust quite particularly that what is happening to me is well done, rightfully done, deemed by God. God in the point, the centre, the heart, of all that is, today. As the needle goes in, as the cannula is flushed, as the healing poison floods my body, God is in all thing.

To the Cancer Village for blood tests four hours before the chemotherapy, to check I'm able to take it. The phlebotomist looks mildly doped, as if she has been up all night partying, but knows what bloods are required and her needle insertion is the best yet — I hardly feel a thing, and certainly no pain.

Then to the dentist high up in Guy's Tower to make sure my teeth are sound before treatment starts. They are.

My bloods pass muster too. I'm in a fit state to receive the poison. Two hours to go.

Seán and I make our way to the Cancer Village in good time for the 3.00pm infusion.

I've been inaccurate in my nomenclature. There are several villages in the Cancer Centre. The Welcome Village, where I check in like an old pro now, then up in the birdsong lift to the Chemotherapy Village. And there's a Radiology Village, and an Outpatient Village, and a Private Treatment Village with carpets, perhaps.

It is quieter up here in the Chemotherapy Village but my heart, which is thumping, briefly fails at the sight of the other patients, those among whom I now count myself, some of them really obviously unwell, creeping with sticks (myeloma?? It's the bones that go) or wheeled in wheelchairs, their faces grey or yellow; the face of the lady in the wheelchair who comes up in the lift with us is worn out, her eyes closing with weariness. And there is an atmosphere of quiet resignation among those waiting, not happy. We sit near the window, away from the other patients, and look at the view, taking in the light and air. Seán notices the word 'mother' in the middle of the word 'chemotherapy' and we are heartened by that, and think we will call the Chemotherapy Village mothercare. But then we are scolded by Deniz, the nurse, because she hasn't found me among the patients outside Suite A, when it is time for me to come in.

So I am a bit flustered, an immediately infantilised patient not wanting to keep the nurse waiting, when I go in and another nurse briskly says 'I've kept seat six for you'. I look around, bewildered, at what at first impression is a combination of three implausible scenes: a pedicure salon with those seats that massage your back while you have your feet done, occupied by the most unlikely clientele; an airport waiting area for first-class passengers because the seats are so big with spaces between them, only the passengers aren't smart business people; and the lounge in a care home. Then I see a big '6' above one of the squashy bright purple pedicure chairs and go and sit in it, still shocked that I am a protagonist here: the seat is for me; I am ill.

I am left alone for a while and I take in my surroundings. There are two large bays; each with a row of three big squishy purple chairs facing each other. I can't see the bay behind me but wonder if that is where the worse patients are treated; I see a man, bald as a coot, wheeled into it in his bed. Is my bay that of the walking wounded perhaps. Opposite me a man, whom I immediately label a gorblimey South London taxi driver, quietly fills in the crossword; his gaunt figure and big eyes and baldish head and his hacking cough are dispiriting. He doesn't return my smile, just glances briefly, then returns to his newspaper. Next to him a middle-aged man has his feet up on the leg rest of the chair (seeing this, I find the zapper and put my leg rest up too: very comfortable and squishy), and shifts restlessly, watching something on his phone; his companion sits, passive, next to him. Later he goes to sleep and loudly snores. In the corner a jolly family, the man in the squishy chair, his daughter (I think) and his wife with him. Everyone is attached to a drip stand with an ominous silver plastic sheath over whatever is in the bag dripping into them. Then a younger, more sprightly man comes in, dressed for work, bearded and with plenty of hair on his head, and is greeted like an old friend: 'You can have either of those seats, R'. He looks like a civil servant. He is hooked up efficiently and starts working on his laptop. After about three-quarters of an hour his drip has finished, the nurse detaches it, and he leaves. He might have been coming in for a haircut.

Nurse Jing comes to set me up. Tut-tut, my veins are not at all satisfactory. Nothing on the right arm, something on the left. 'I will be gentle,' she says. She will use the smallest needle. In the cannula goes, just below my left hand. It hurts but is comfortable enough once in. Then she sets up a small drip, a saline solution to flush out the cannula. 'Can I go to the loo?' I ask anxiously. 'Oh yes,' she says. 'Just unplug your drip at the wall and take it with you.' That seems a tall order, but I see Mr Gaunt opposite me do it, so it must be possible. 'Some patients are infused for seven hours,' says nurse Jing. 'Of course they have to go to the loo.'

Soon after, nurse Deniz appears. She gives me my two Dexamethasone tablets, 40mg of steroids which will probably keep me awake tonight. Kind to give them as early as possible; in future I can take them myself early in the morning. She changes the flushing-out drip bag for the hydration drip bag. I have to have extra hydration before and after Carfilzomib in my first cycle of chemotherapy to help me tolerate its onslaught. It will take half an hour, says Deniz: relax. I haven't, at all, up until this point. I open Alexander McCall Smith's *44 Scotland Street*, written episodically as that was how it was published in a daily newspaper, with each short chapter a mercifully engaging vignette, making me laugh out loud, even now. I love him.

Then. The Carfilzomib. Swiftly, briskly, but carefully set up by two nurses double checking the process. My name and date of birth asked for again. My hospital number read out, the bag hung from the drip machine, the silver plastic sheath over the bag now sporting a 'released' label, connected to the cannula in my wrist, and I am off. For all the drama I have built up in my mind, for all my intention to receive the chemotherapy consciously, imagining my body porously receiving it, accepting it as treatment and not rejecting it, the fact is that at this moment I desperately need a pee, so I have to get up, unplug the drip, and make my way unsteadily to the mercifully prox-imate lavatory. I don't swoon or feel sick. I feel spaced out but that could just be the weird situation I am in.

When I sit down again, I meditate and go all internally receptive. A's words, you told me you said before you were anaesthetised for your heart bypass operation, sound in my heart: 'Father, into thy hands I commend my spirit'(Luke 23:46, KJV). The half hour passes quickly. Then another half an hour of hydration, to help my body receive the Carfilzomib. 'You have tolerated it well,' says nurse Deniz, approvingly, as she changes the bags. Infantile still, I am glad, want-ing to please Deniz, but of course I am also dripping (ha) with relief that I haven't reacted badly.

While I am hydrating, Seán comes in, sporting a bright green shiny windmill which spins as he blows on it. My surprise treat for getting through the ordeal. Everyone smiles, and as he sits down our corner fills with laughter. I need the loo again and do a little dance with my drip as I make my way, saying 'After you' before wheeling it into the lavatory cubicle, and getting the drip line and the plug cable tangled up so I have to be disentangled by nurse Jing on my return.

Nurse Deniz comes up with a HUGE bag of pharmaceuticals. From one of the pile of boxes she tips ten Cyclophosphomide tablets (also chemotherapy) into a little cup for me to swallow then and there, and going through all the others, those I had to take one of once a day before breakfast (Omeprazole, stomach liner); those of which I had to take one, twice a day (Ciprofloxacin, antibiotic and Aciclovir, antiviral); those of which I had to take three, once a day (Allopurinol, kidney protection) and, because I check my list and she hasn't included them, and I know they were on it, Domperidone, anti-sickness, to be taken when needed. 'Dom Perignon', says Deniz. 'Don't take them unless you need to because you don't want to reduce their efficacy by overuse.' Could the same be true of champagne?

I totter home with Seán, light-headed and shaky, but mostly with relief. I want, quite specifically, primavera risotto and salad for supper, not too much, lots more water, and a long soak in an Epsom salt bath.

Friday, 3 May

I don't feel sick. I am alive.

The night is all right. Not only do I neither vomit nor want to vomit, I sleep quite well, despite the steroids that I had only taken at 3.30pm. However. An early discovery when I return this morning for my next infusion, and am given two more steroid tablets, is that they are not the massive dose of Dexamethasone I think they are, but only a little pre-med dose given before each infusion to help it along. I have failed – already! – to take my weekly, massive dose of Dexamethasone. So I have to do it straightaway, special permission from Grace given over the phone since I am a day late and I am on the Cardamon trial and nothing should be done off-protocol. Seán has to bring the bottle of Dexamethasone tablets specially from the flat for me. Now I can't remember if nurse Deniz had, in fact, given them to me when she gave me my first weekly dose of Cyclophosphamide yesterday, when I was obediently swallowing everything I was given, like an infant. Nurse Jing gives us a little tray and two pots and Seán and I are tasked with counting the pills. There will be eighty tablets in the bottle if I have not taken my dose; sixty if I have. There are seventy-nine. We panic. Seán confesses that the lid was not fastened when he took the bottle from the special place I had assigned it in a kitchen cupboard and the pills had scattered all over the counter. Perhaps one has fallen to the floor and rolled under the washing machine. Nurse Jing has to phone Grace again and ask if she can add another tablet to our store. Meanwhile I swallow twenty tablets, each 2mg. Twenty!

This is my second visit and I am already more confident and connected to my fellow patients, smiling sympathetically at the new ones waiting nervously to be called, looking with interest at who my neighbours are when I enter Suite A again, knowing how to arrange the squishy purple chair to my comfort, getting out my book, greeting nurse Jing like an old friend . . . Oh how quickly we habituate ourselves. This is my new normal.

When Jing searches for a vein for my Friday infusion she fails in her first attempt. It hurts. I am to ask Grace if I can have a port line fitted, which sounds like something one would use to ensure one's levels of Cockburn are kept topped up, but isn't. It's a 'portable catheter', a little plastic device placed under the skin about where the Queen's brooches sit on her coat, only on the right-hand side, and you can keep it in for up to five years. Since I'll be receiving Carfilzomib, on and off, for the next two years, it makes sense. And everything can be done with it: blood taking, drip giving. 'No more needles,' says Jing brightly. Yet another way in which I will become a long-term patient, something of which I am only too well-reminded when I take my raft of drugs in the morning. I should get one of those pill dispensers with the days of the week and the times of the day . . . but, oh dear, the thought of it does make me feel geriatric.

There are more and different patients today. One lady has on, I think, one of those cold caps recommended if you're having chemotherapy that makes your hair fall out. It looks like the bonnet rugby players wear. Hard to bear if it's really cold and your infusion is a long one, but worth it, I'm certain. Then the lady on my left shows me her beautiful, bald head. She looks exhausted. Years of chemotherapy; a double mastectomy; big eyes; resignation. The lady on my right is similarly a years-long patient, brightly accepting that she can't have her infusion today as her temperature is too high. Opposite, an Italian man speaks too loudly into his phone: 'They couldn't finda my fucking vein'. A Spanish (I think) lady is next to him, speaking quietly to her companion. Then a tall lady comes in to the corner seat where R sat yesterday: she is well dressed and efficient, carefully removing her jacket and folding it, sitting down, knowing what to do: she looks like a civil servant too.

I feel proud to be included among this diverse mix of companions in mothercare. This is my cancer gang.

My treatment complete, Seán and I make our way straight to London Bridge station to catch a train to Hastings. On the platform I − now − notice several women with headscarves and no eyelashes. We all totter from treatment to train to home and rest. It is strangely marvellous to be here.

Saturday, 4 May

Today a healing massage and sacro-cranial treatment from Samvida, in her cottage buried in rural Sussex, then communing with her horses and a walk in the woods. I am alone in the woods for a while, sobbing. Down from the steroid high, perhaps, but I need to cry. I am all right, I feel all right, but this is sad and hard. It's going to go on for a long time, and I am having to focus so carefully on myself, taking prescribed drugs at prescribed times, careful not to catch any infection (I have masks now, and I wear them in enclosed spaces like the cinema or the car with my friends), I can't be thoughtless. I'm not sick but I feel full of strange substances and my stomach is particular. A tentative glass of wine, some lamb, litres and litres of water. But the tears which are for sadness become, after a while, tears of gratitude. I am standing in the most beautiful copse, the bluebells still making their hazy carpet under old silver birches, the birds chirping, the sunlight dappling through the new green leaves. It is, truly, beautiful. I weep for beauty. I thank God for beauty.

And when I go to see the horses again before returning to Sam's cottage, standing at the gate of their enclosure, BJ the big horse with a blaze on his nose comes over to me. He takes a long time to do it, swaying his head, but I somehow know he is coming, and wait. He makes me cry all over again. He has cancer too.

Sixth Letter

Dear Readers

F, thank you for quoting Gerard Manley Hopkins' 'Pied Beauty', one of our favourite poems. It suits the mood of gratitude in the wood last Saturday, for the transient perfection of what was shown and for the fecund unceasing love that showed it:

> With swift, slow; sweet, sour; adazzle, dim;
> He fathers-forth whose beauty is past change:
> Praise him.[1]

And for George Herbert's 'The Temper (I)', especially the last stanza, J, that helped you when you had cancer treatment and now helps me:

> Whether I fly with angels, fall with dust,
> Thy hands made both, and I am there;
> Thy power and love, my love and trust
> Make one place ev'ry where.[2]

I feel amazingly well. Fraudulently fit. Not just physically fit but filled with well-being and my skin glows with health (it must be all that water). M and I go for a stroll along the river from Borough Market to Tate Modern, across the wobbly bridge to St Paul's and back again to the flat. Seán works with our dear friend A to set up a new TV and, novices to Netflix, we start to watch *The Crown* that evening, speaking to each other in clipped accents afterwards. Cancer and all its attendant woes recede. But then I think: I feel normal so I should be in the office.

Julian's revelations take place on a crucifix her curate is holding before her eyes as she lies, apparently dying, in bed; it is this crucifix that she sees move and speak and bleed. In her fourth vision blood flows from the crucifix in abundance, not only over all the Earth but also down into hell and up into heaven where Christ still bleeds for humanity. Julian thinks of all the water in the world God has made available for human use; but of the blood, she sees, 'there is no liquor that he liketh so well to give us, for it is most plenteous as it is most precious'. Water washes us but Christ's blood *really* washes us, inside and out. Of our sins.

I am not a good Christian. I would far rather wash in water than in blood. Less sticky. And sin is a hard word to hear. When I was environmental adviser to the Church of England we said that pollution was a sin. The mischievous *Sunday Times* created a front-page headline: 'Bishop says flying is a sin', and an unexpectedly raw nerve was touched. For a week we were interviewed by furious news journalists: how dare we say people are sinners.

But it seems to me that without a sense of sin — I mean proper moral responsibility — there can be no remorse and without remorse there can be no melting of the heart, no possibility of porosity to the other, of accepting help.

I do not think that cancer is a punishment for my sins. Never that. Never, ever that. But I do think this: I fully share responsibility for the overall mess that humans generally make of our world, cancer being a still largely unexplained part of that mess; I am sorry; I accept that I cannot, on my own, make reparation or make good; I accept help. And (this is strangely hard to write) forgiveness.

That, at any rate, is my aspiration. Dear E, your fury at Seán's and my undeserved misfortune can abate. Bad things happen to all of us, and we're in it together, we're not more or less deserving than each other.

Today, this is how I receive and understand and accept Julian's blood–flood. There is so much water and blood in my life now: three litres of water to be drunk throughout each day; phials of blood withdrawn every week from the crook of my elbow; bleeding into the cannula to ensure the nurse has found a vein to infuse the Carfilzomib and then infuse more water for hydration; and every day the recollection, sometimes through deliberate gentle meditation, of the blood flowing throughout my body, bringing life and also producing the cells that will harm me. Blood and water mixed like the blood-of-Christ wine and water mixed in the eucharistic chalice. They pass through my body, washing me deep inside, flowing through arteries and veins and capillaries, even into my very marrow where the cancer is active. A sacred symphony to heal my helpless self. I am made porous by humility and I hear the symphony and I am grateful.

Thursday, 9 May

Waiting in mothercare to be called in for my infusion, I think: Thank God I have no children. And I think: Maybe I didn't have children because our mother died of cancer when we were still children and, consciously or unconsciously, I couldn't risk a repeat abandonment. Maybe that is one of the reasons. Well here I am at fifty-four and there can, now, be no repeat, but is that a good thing?

Oh, I am touched by my fellow humans here.

The man in front of me, resting his elbows on the table and his face in his hands, his beanie pushed to the back of his not-hairless head. What is he feeling?

The heartfelt thank-you cards stuck to the wall behind the receptionists' desk.

The big fat lady with the jolly face and spectacles going back and forth with great swag bags of our drugs from pharmacy to chemotherapy suites, so we don't have to.

The brave dignity of patients walking out of suites with their heads held high, quietly, often slowly, or firmly, like the grey-haired man making his way to the stairs just now, eyes fixed on the path ahead of him. His carer (wife?), walking just behind him, has hunched shoulders by contrast, her eyes darting anxiously from him to the nurses to the tea station to the stairs: what else can I do, what is required of me now? The patient is calm and focused on his one single worry.

A man in a red cap and red shoes with a strong voice argues on the phone with what must be a housing officer: repairs are needed in his house. Maybe it's a distraction but who here needs the additional worry of things going wrong at home?

There's a long delay this afternoon. Plenty of nurses, plenty of drugs, but no spare purple squashy chairs. One in, one out. Everyone's regime is different and some are in there for the day. Finally I am called. As I settle myself in the purple squish, a very tall, thin Black man walks past, with a bright sequined cap on, accompanied by several tall Black women: they look like the gods of Arcadia passing by.

In the chair opposite me a woman is scrolling on her phone, her comments indicating she is looking at wigs and hats. Her hair looks abundant: a tumble of golden curls, but she is upbeat, really liking this look, not so much that one, ooh this would be nice. Her bright and matter-of-fact attention to the options for baldness is beautiful. Later we talk and I learn she has children and grandchildren, though she looks quite young. She has pancreatic cancer, and her treatment is horrendous: fifty-six hours of infusion beginning in the chair here and carrying on with a pump at home; while it is going on she can hardly get out of bed she feels so ill with it. An endurance test repeated every fortnight, for six months. Her mother is with her. They are positive. 'You have to do it for the children,' she says. She took the risk of having children and they will help her endure the course.

The young man in the corner chair is shivering under a blanket with a hot pad held to his front. He retches and coughs. The large man in the chair next to me is bald; his face is like a child's, his movements slow.

We are all troubling to stay alive.

Friday, 10 May

In mothercare for the second infusion of the week, I watch a lady being given a gentle oily massage into her hair before a cold cap is fastened on her head. I think the caps feel very cold but she is clearly habituated, resigned. Her veins aren't being amenable to the cannula's needle and she has to wait while a warm pad hopefully brings them out to play.

Today I am tired, I can't think of words, miscount my pills, am constipated, seem to be having a double dose of hot flushes. Of course this is the day after my massive dose of Dexamethasone (steroid) and I can expect to feel depressed. But my blood pressure is amazing; it's never been this good. It's all the fluid, says the nurse. I'm briefly furious with kidney Dr Adam. He would have put me on blood pressure tablets for the rest of my life to control my kidneys' raised creatinine (when we thought that was the problem, before myeloma raised its bloody head). Why couldn't he prescribe three litres of water a day? Which would you rather?

When we were small an absolute favourite pastime was dancing with our aunt to the song about Lily the Pink and her 'Medicinal Compound'.[3] The 'most efficacious' tonic turns out to be water and I suppose this was an early introduction to irony, but my beautician confirms that it's the best medicine for loads of things: skin, hair, weight, blood pressure, bloating . . . I rest my case, Dr Adam.

Above the doors into the chemotherapy suite is a sign which reads 'Acute Chemotherapy'. But surely chemotherapy for myeloma is palliative, I think, until a cure is found? But the name above the door makes me think: 'They want me to live.'

I feel a fraud. Most of all I feel undeserving. It may be my psyche's Dexamethasone descent but I do feel undeserving. I just do. Why on Earth should I be kept alive when millions aren't?

I am given a squashy chair by the window and am calmed by the views over south London while the infusions take place. The cannula finds a home first go. And we are quick to catch a train to Hastings; I drink in gratefully the exquisite views of rolling hills and spring-green trees and blackthorn bud bursts through Kent and Sussex and I don't feel too sick.

Sunday, 12 May

Saturday. Was. Shit.

I wasn't actually sick (burp not retch, thank God) but I was in that awful no-man's-land of not knowing if I was nauseous or hungry. I had appointments for a pedicure and a facial, both of which seemed excellent ideas at the time, and, madly, I struggled out of bed and kept them. They were endurance tests as the wafty smells of aromatherapy became, for me, aroma-sickly-sweetness. Afterwards I could only lie on the sofa and gently moan, dutifully swallowing my drugs and my water, finally taking a Domperidone for sickness in the afternoon though it didn't seem to make much difference. I read the gently humorous and utterly comforting *Oldie* from cover to cover.

Now I am writing about it the feeling of nauseousness is coming back. Steady the buffs. Deep breaths. There. It's gone. I'll have breakfast. I have energy.

But oh no! I wash my hair and more than just one or two strands come out, and more come out as I comb it too. Not many, not so's you'd notice, but some.

Another verse from George Herbert's 'The Temper' (thank you, J):

> Yet take thy way; for sure thy way is best:
> Stretch or contract me, thy poor debtor:
> This is but tuning of my breast,
> To make the music better.[4]

Consent to be stretched, Claire.

Seán thinks I'll reveal a lovely shaped egghead under my hair.

Seventh Letter

Dear Readers

I seek to tune in to God with very, very quiet listening. I consent to be stretched. I face the confounding work of chemotherapy: to make the body receive and not resist. I have to let the poisonous healing get the better of me so I cannot brace myself against it, but I do not have to shrink and be weak. I can come positively and intentionally face to face with it, and say 'yes' to it with strength in my voice and my heart.

Thursday, 16 May

Thursdays are complicated.

I wake early and go to the kitchen to take the twenty tablets, 2mg each, of the steroid Dexamethasone. As early as possible because it's a big dose and will keep me awake tonight. I put the first five tablets in my mouth, then remember I need to eat first, and carefully eject them into the lid of the pill bottle. I bite on a banana, then remember that I have to take the stomach-lining drug Omeprazole before eating. I stand paralysed by my dilemma: do I spit out the banana too and go and take Omeprazole (I keep it by my bed) first? But the Dexamethasone tablets are gently fizzing and starting to dissolve and possibly won't wait for me to go back on myself. I'm meant to leave half an hour between Omeprazole and Dexamethasone. So I eat the banana, swallow the twenty tablets, and go back to bed, thinking I will start the day again later with Omeprazole. Even though the Omeprazole is to stop the Dexamethasone hurting my stomach . . .

After lying and not sleeping for a while, breakfast, but that involves milk, and the kidney drugs should be taken at least two hours after milk, but not too late as they are taken with the other drugs (antiviral, antibiotic), and *they* are taken twice a day so there has to be enough of a gap between the morning ones and the evening ones.

(I have succumbed to a pill box.)

So: breakfast not too late; drugs two hours later; then into the Cancer Centre for blood tests which have to be done three hours before the Carfilzomib infusion to give the pharmacy time to make the drug up. It's 3.30pm for the Carfilzomib so 11.00am, to be safe, for the blood tests.

Then remembering to take the Cyclophosphamide tablets with me to the Cancer Centre at 3.30pm. I ask the nurse to give me these because they are so poisonous they can't be touched and I am afraid I'll mess up, drop them or something. I feel the nurses need to take care of such poison; they know how.

Supposing I had a family to look after or a job that had demanded I still be present and functioning? Suppose I had *anything* else to organise apart from those pills and the combination of visits, every week slightly different? It is a full-time job. By which I mean it has to be the priority in my thinking and planning and everything else has to fit in around it. Suppose I had even one thing that was dependent upon me and also demanded priority attention? Most people do.

Today my phlebotomist, Joachim, is an unsmiling ten-year-old (to my eyes). Without warning, in goes the needle for the blood test, bloody painful, but extremely quick.

Today when I come for the infusion in the afternoon, I employ an Ignatian technique: I invite Jesus into mothercare. More than that, I imagine him entering my body with the Carfilzomib. Into my body he flows, through my poor battered veins, with the healing poison, going to meet the cancer in my very marrow.

A lady opposite is on the phone, rather too loudly for my comfort, but she is desperately worried about someone who is in terrible pain at home and is not being attended to. She makes several phone calls, and eventually it seems the matter is resolved. She is not young; she has myeloma, I gather from earwigging, which manifested first for her as chest pains that took for ever to diagnose, pains that were so bad she couldn't lie on her side.

So again I am made grateful for my lot. Early diagnosis: no symptoms, no pain except now from the treatment. A calm domestic scene with no demands on my attention. A job I am able to keep. A home by the sea in which to recover from side effects. Most valuable and wondrous gift of all: a beautiful man to care for me.

Friday, 17 May

Oh Lord, it is hard again.

I can't walk too quickly after chemotherapy: it makes me feel ill, as though the poison is sloshing through my body. I collapse on the stairs at home, sobbing with relief that I'm not going to have to have an infusion for nearly a fortnight, my poor bruised forearms with the evidence of failed and successful attempts to get the cannulas in; tender swollen veins where the Carfilzomib has irritated them; unsmiling Joachim's blood-taking puncture still angry red and I feel sick. I feel sick.

I don't want this. I want it to stop. I'm not strong or positive or learning anything or seeing any point. I'm just sick: vulnerable, unhappy, raw, weak. Weak!

Saturday, 18 May

I determine that I am all right, I don't feel sick, just a little unsettled. Then I give in, and realise I do feel sick. So then I take a Domperidone pill. Admit you're not well, then you can accept help. But now the braced, positive feeling in me that makes me strong and able to cope has gone. Now I am helpless and vulnerable, an ill person. I have surrendered my autonomy. I know in theory, and indeed theologically, the value of this: I wasn't autonomous to begin with; we all deeply depend upon each other; none of us can manage on our own; I am arrogant if I think I can; but I DO NOT want to be a passenger. I become so unsure of myself when I cannot help myself. I don't like relinquishing control.

This is the truth of it: I'm not sure if anyone will like me, just as I am.

Sunday, 19 May

I make it to the second half of mass and receive a blessing from Fr Eamonn, who is himself struck low by the death of a dear friend. He speaks about the importance of grief. I haven't tried to cheer myself up today; I haven't tried to do anything about anything, just cry a bit and read the papers and play solitaire and help Seán water the garden at the back.

And now I'm writing this, sitting at the table, looking out over the sea and the houses of the Old Town, nestling between the West Hill where I am and the East Hill across the valley. The houses look like what they once were, medieval dwellings jumbled together, roofs of different pitch and colour. The green of the hill behind forms a protecting embrace. The sea is blue–grey. A pigeon perches on an aerial and a blackbird warbles the evening in. I can feel my sense of humour stealing back. We shall have pasta tonight.

Eighth Letter

Dear Readers

I need that sense of humour. This morning does not bring physical relief. I'm not sick, just weary, and headachy; the weather is lowering as if a storm is brewing and it feels hard to breathe. No energy. But I feel obligated. I have to pull myself together, find my energy from motivation if not from my body, because I have to go to London for some final Institute meetings. How often have I relied on that brittle energy! I am pulling at my old self, the one I relied upon to deliver, no matter what my physical state. Come on Claire, up you get, out you go. But I can't. I lie in bed, mentally beating myself up.

> My own heart let me more have pity on . . .
> With this tormented mind tormenting yet.
> I cast for comfort I can no more get . . .[5]

I accept that I don't feel well and I cancel the London meetings. Now I need to take my temperature. This is a moment of decision: if I have a temperature of 37.5 degrees or above, I have to ring the emergency helpline number and in all probability go to hospital, because a high temperature usually means infection and in the absence of a functioning immune system an infection could be lethal. I do not want to go to hospital. Oh, Dear Readers, the nonsense reasoning I go through. I will only have a high temperature if I take it. It will go away if I don't look. And then I won't have to go to hospital.

I look and it is high: 38.2 degrees. The helpline nurse tells me to go to hospital. The Conquest in Hastings has a perfectly pleasant A & E department; at 1.00pm it's not busy though one of the patients is quietly accompanied by a police escort. I am seen immediately (everyone else is taking this seriously), have 'me vitals' taken (blood pressure 180 over something, bloody hell) and am ushered into a cupboard and on to a trolley. Also squeezed into the cupboard are a desk and a chair, on which Seán sits. He gazes at a small piece of carrot shrivelling on the desk top as the nurse assures us the room has been deep-cleaned. Another nurse takes some blood and inserts a cannula. Then another nurse hooks me up to drips with paracetamol and an antibiotic, given prophylactically, before the blood tests checking the presence of infection are complete: no risks taken. We chemotherapy junkies have to have antibiotics within four hours of gaining an infection to be safe. 'Oh darling you'll be in overnight,' says this nurse. 'Although your lactation test is good.' Seán and I are certain that that is what she says. 'And you're not pregnant.' There's a relief. I am wheeled out for a chest x-ray. 'Are you pregnant?' asks the radiologist, who could be a carbon copy of the beautiful young radiologist at Guy's. Afterwards I am wheeled back to my cupboard. Another nurse comes in and says 'Beef bourgignon; cod mornay; macaroni cheese.' My swift to make sense — the wrong sense — of this theatre of the absurd has me assuming he is asking me to tell him which of those dishes my symptoms most resemble. Perhaps I am a little delirious. The thing is, everyone is wearing blue pyjamas, so how is one to realise their different functions? This is the caterer and I have to choose a dish for . . . it is 3.00pm. Supper? I choose with a sinking heart: doing so is tantamount to accepting that I will be staying the night. I have realised that the cupboard I am in isn't a holding bay, though I am on a trolley. It is a room in the A & E ward, and the shared smelly loo with a shower behind a thin curtain across the way will be my ablution station.

I have another visitor in blue pyjamas, but luckily he identifies himself as a doctor. He looks extremely young. He listens to various things with his stethoscope and taps other things, asks me how I feel. 'Fine,' I insist, glaring at Seán when he starts to tell the doctor about my cough. He says he'll be back when the blood test results are through.

Seán and I read our books. I try not to worry about my sleeping arrangements. The trolley has just a single sheet on it, already blood-stained (with my blood) and is slipping off the slippery surface.

But sooner than we could have hoped, the doctor returns. 'The blood tests are all right,' he says. 'You can go home. In the nicest possible way, I hope I don't see you again.'

> . . . let joy size
> At God knows when to God knows what; whose smile
> 's not wrung, see you; unforeseen times rather — as skies
> Betweenpie mountains — lights a lovely mile.[6]

Tuesday, 21 May

Today I wake to a brave new world, my bursting appreciation matching the depth of my earlier despairing nausea and fever (does one have to have the ghastliness before one can have the joy?). The lowering skies have lifted, the sun shines on a glittering sea, the smell of summer is everywhere. Today I ride and I don't think I have the words to express how joyful that feels. My lovely friends at the stables couldn't have been kinder, adding me to the hack at the last minute. 'It's what we can do to help,' says Rachel. I ride big, strong Denby, sturdy as a mountain, and drink in all of nature: rolling hills, abundant oaks, ancient beech, a buzzard hovering, wending our way through overgrown paths and cantering along the trampoline field and the uppy-downy field, birdsong, the smells richer than I have ever known them. And as we return, I see you, M, waiting to bring me home, sitting sketching two ponies who have come close to you, out of curiosity maybe, and are grazing at your feet.

It is the opposite of a hospital, where nothing green grows (except culture on the bit of carrot, maybe). The warmth there is human kindness.

Wednesday, 22 May

The nausea returns after yesterday's 'lovely mile', and stays with me until bedtime. What a bloody awful week so far.

Thursday, 23 May

Julian's sixth revelation is one in which she sees how God worships and thanks those who seek to serve him in their lives. 'The more that the loving soul seeth this courtesy of God, the lever he is to serve him all the dayes of his life.' I try to turn my sickness to service. 'Offer it up,' I hear you say, P. And as I write this now, I do, with all my heart. But only afterwards: while I feel ill, I am helpless, inert, without motive or motion. Desolate.

Today (week off – no chemotherapy!) I revel in the lack of nausea, and the euphoria and appetite the high Dexamethasone dose – still have to take my steroids – gives me. L and I go for a walk; I vote; buy olive oil; and in the evening Seán and I, masked, go to the dance interpretation of T.S. Eliot's *Four Quartets* at the Barbican. I love hearing the poems read and the accompanying music; the dance is sometimes wonderful and sometimes distracting, mainly because I am trying to understand what the choreography means, and of course the dancers keep moving and you don't have time to linger on one step or shape and think about it. You have to let go and follow, let it work on you.

The words move fast too, but you can return to the words.

Friday, 24 May

I have my end-of-cycle appointment with the consultant: beautiful articulate Dr Reuben. He tells me to take the Domperidone prophylactically. 'If you are too nauseous we will have to stop the chemotherapy.' I ask for a port because of my cannula challenges but he is strangely resistant and makes no commitment. He tells me the likely outcome of my treatment: I have a seventy to eighty per cent chance of 'good remission', which means the numbers of kappa light chains and paraproteins are halved. Keeping the numbers down means keeping the cancer symptoms at bay. With incurable myeloma, that is the most you can hope for.

I will have the results showing how I have responded to my first cycle of chemotherapy next week.

I ask about stem cell harvesting, which everyone in the trial goes through, even if they don't have the stem cell transplant, because the stem cells can be used for a later transplant if you need one. Answer: I will have a big dose of chemotherapy, then growth factor injections in my stomach every day for a week, then at least five hours hooked up to a machine which takes my blood away and gives it back to me with (hopefully) lots of stem cells removed.

You can know things, and you can know things more fully, and you can know things even more fully. Today I feel I know even more fully that I have cancer, and when I go to bed, I clutch my rosary to my breast and sob. I can't pray or think or make sense or rationalise or sort anything out. I just feel. Pain. And then I fall asleep.

Thank you, M, for sending this; the poetry articulates my grief relieved only by sleep:

> No worst, there is none. Pitched past pitch of grief,
> More pangs will, schooled at forepangs, wilder wring.
> Comforter, where, where is your comforting?
> Mary, mother of us, where is your relief?
> My cries heave, herds-long; huddle in a main, a chief
> Woe, wórld-sorrow; on an áge-old anvil wince and sing –
> Then lull, then leave off. Fury had shrieked 'No ling-
> ering! Let me be fell: force I must be brief.'
>
> O the mind, mind has mountains; cliffs of fall
> Frightful, sheer, no-man-fathomed. Hold them cheap
> May who ne'er hung there. Nor does long our small
> Durance deal with that steep or deep. Here! creep,
> Wretch, under a comfort serves in a whirlwind: all
> Life death does end and each day dies with sleep.[7]

Sunday, 26 May

This Will Not Do. I am strong and I am surrounded by people who not only want me to live, but also know the best possible way to make that happen. The least I can do is cheer up and take the medicine with a smile. I've been through one cycle now. I can do this.

I bathe in scented salts, don a voluptuous heavy silk kaftan, pour delicate Wraxall's pink sparkling wine into a champagne glass, and dress my hair. And put on bright orange lipstick. Very seventies and I feel much better.

Thank you, L, who also bounced around the room with us to 'Lily the Pink' as small children, for the information that the real Lily the Pink was an American woman called Lydia Pinkham (1819–83) who invented a 'herbal-alcoholic women's tonic', probably mainly gin, available during Prohibition and hence immensely popular. So not water at all. We wuz lied to.

Ninth Letter

Dear Readers

I am grieving. Without the motivation of work or other external demands I am thrown into a new and strange space. I really do only have to be concerned with taking the drugs, drinking the water, turning up for appointments, receiving the chemotherapy. Yes, I can work at home, and I am really glad to have research and writing to do, but it is not my priority and no one is drumming their fingers waiting for it. No one is depending upon me. There's no 'show-time', as you would say, J, to ready myself for, no curtain rising on an expectant audience looking to me for a performance.

An enforced sabbatical, a real sabbath, a long one. I pray it is transformative. Sometimes I feel comforted, sometimes I don't, but I do not doubt that Love is constant. May it 'wash me throughly' (Psalm 51:2, KJV).

Tuesday, 28 May

Another glorious ride on Denby. His canter is quite exciting because although he has this quality of mountain-like strength that makes me feel utterly supported, he is fast and powerful and you sense that in the canter: a physical prowess that is quite beyond my experience, I can only feel it, respect it, ride it. And then just quietly walking: to see the rolling countryside – the rich, bursting-forth greenness of it, the distant sea shimmering, the light – from the back of a horse is a grand privilege. I feel nurtured by the horse. Through my connection with him I am drawn into nature's warp and weft.

68

Wednesday, 29 May

A singing lesson! What joy! Riding, singing: these experiences seem richer, my gratitude deeper, because of the cancer. I wouldn't wish it on anyone but look at the new depths it is giving me.

My greatest challenge is to allow, let be. Let the treatment work. Beloved J, asking me to sleep, and to let all of you carry me in your prayers (and equivalent for those of you who would not call it prayer). I have never done this before! To trust myself to others so completely. Not to try to make myself pleasing to God, or to demand anything of myself. To let be. Let be.

Thursday, 30 May

Cycle two starts today, with its complicated dance of drug-taking, blood-letting and chemotherapy-infusing. But in the evening, a phone call from Grace with one of the results showing how I have responded to the first cycle of treatment. It is startling.

A normal person will have somewhere between three and nineteen kappa light chains. When I started treatment I had 1,102. I now have . . . fourteen!!

So obviously, I want to stop everything. I almost don't have cancer anymore and I can go back to not having to go to hospital all the time and take all these drugs.

No, says Grace, her voice kind. You carry on with the treatment, to the end.

Of course. I still have cancer and I will always have cancer. And I haven't had all the results. But how cheering to see such a response already. It does help my feelings towards the chemotherapy.

Friday, 31 May

After the treatment, straight out of Guy's and on to a train at London Bridge. A long journey to Hastings, the restorative countryside view from the train easing my queasiness. I collapse in bed and sleep, utterly relieved to be here. When I awaken the sun has emerged, reflected in the jumble of houses of the Old Town; the sea is calm, and I feel a bit better.

And then in the evening another phone call from Grace with the other result: my paraprotein level has halved from eleven to six. (Normal people don't have any paraproteins.) This is, as Grace says, very good news indeed. It confirms that the treatment is working.

Bless you, team at Guy's, Matthew, Mary, Grace, Sarah, Deniz, Jing, Joachim (even) and all of you whose names I don't know yet. Bless you Carfilzomib, Cyclophosphamide and Dexamethasone.

I feel rotten tonight. But this hard-to-endure treatment is made so much easier to bear when it shows a response.

Saturday, 1 June

Nausea day again, but I think it isn't as bad as before. I'm not entirely incapacitated, not actually queasy except in horrid waves that come but also go; I am able to eat a little. And a wonderful present, thank you N: a painting-by-numbers set. Perfect for nausea days. Once again, I am carried; someone else has done all the work; I just have to colour in the shapes. It is like being prayed for. Inspired by the notion, I also start a jigsaw puzzle of a Roman mosaic.

Sunday, 2 June

At mass Fr Eamonn, whom I adore anyway but particularly because he always introduces a period of silence at the end of his homilies, asks us to consider, in that silence, what is life-giving to us. I immediately start thinking of what I think I ought to find life-giving, instead of what I actually find life-giving. And I realise I don't really know. That's not completely true, of course: I know that Seán's company is life-giving; singing and riding are life-giving; writing is life-giving, and so is P.G. Wodehouse and so are Jeremy Hardy's monologues; but deep within me, in my very heart . . .? I feel there *is* an answer to this question but I have to wait and listen some more, and give myself plenty of time to find the words, and I think that words may never be enough to articulate the answer.

Because myeloma is incurable, the good results from the first cycle of treatment are immensely cheering but they do not signify to me the winning of a battle, or even a successful first skirmish. They mean that we are on the right track, I am in the right place, I have submitted myself to the right regime, and I have been given the best chance to live as long as possible without symptoms.

I think I am better off than if I were to be thinking about my cancer as an enemy to be defeated. I have a benign, resting-with feeling about the myeloma: it's with me and will always be with me, so I cannot hate it because that would mean I would hate a part of myself.

Well now.

I think I am simply realising the human condition: our wounded selves. My wound has a name, myeloma. But I have other wounds too. Disabled people's wounds are obvious, so-called able people's wounds are not; disabled people can teach the apparently able a great deal more than vice versa.

I'm meeting Donald Trump tomorrow.

Tenth Letter

Dear Readers

I have Donald Trump in my nose! Horrified, I sluice and snort in the Dean's lavatory as I try to wash the nasty little Trump cells away. I have carefully not touched any of my beloved colleagues at Westminster Abbey when I join them to greet Mr Trump on his state visit, longing to hug them, so delighted to see everyone, but needing to be careful of infection. But I know I will have to shake Mr Trump's hand and, as it turns out, those of his offspring and the US Ambassador and the Duke of York. Thereafter a thorough hand-washing is needed. In the privacy of the lavatory, without thinking (unpleasant bodily detail coming up), I pick my nose, before I have washed my hands. That's how he gets there. Grace did warn me that I pose the greatest threat of infection to myself.

Wednesday, 5 June

I am counting hairs. It feels rather ridiculous and spectrumy (but I am a bit spectrumy) and then I think of the Sermon on the Mount and how every hair on my head is counted (I think it's in the Sermon on the Mount). So that feels biblical. Yesterday I counted seventy-two in my comb. That feels biblical too, because Jesus sends out seventy-two disciples in the Gospel of Luke. Having counted once I think I had better count today. Ninety-nine hairs. I will have to count again when I next wash my hair, because that's quite a steep rise. And I'll wash my hair less often.

Sunday, 9 June

There is a sailing boat making its way slowly across the calm sea. It is 6.00am, the sun has risen again, and I *feel better*. I weep for gratitude that the world has returned, brought Sunday and me with it, not left me behind, in my miserable, lonely, queasy, useless Saturday. Enraged, by the evening, at the monumental waste of time: a whole day gone, a whole day lost every week to the poisonous healer. This morning, I have a prayer, that these enforced helpless times will be to the good in some way. Now, in this quiet morning moment, I offer them, and my acceptance of them, to God: you will have to make good of them. For the life of me, I do not know how to.

The first time I was invited to go sailing I remember asking what one did during all those hours of idleness as the boat scudded through the waves, drawn by the wind in the sails, in between rare moments of crisis when you think you are going to die. ('Sailing: it's all climax and no foreplay', to misquote Caroline Chartres.) 'Nothing' was the response, but I could not know until I had tried it how full that 'nothing' is, as one simply relaxes and merges into the elements, deeply enjoying their power and one's connection with them. Can I, can I possibly find some parity between that and my helpless nausea? In theory.

In her seventh revelation, Julian of Norwich experiences 'weal and woe' some twenty times. That is, she feels marvellous, full of God's bliss and delight, a 'sovereign ghostly liking in my soul' in one moment, and then immediately afterwards she feels utterly bereft and despairing, in 'heaviness and weariness of my life and irkness of myself'. She moves from the bliss to the pain, back and forth, so swiftly that she knows she had no hand in causing either state. I think of yesterday's pointless woe and today's undeserved weal. 'Both is one love,' she reflects.

The gulls have nested again on our roof. Previously worried about letting them (why?), for the last two years we have been more concerned about gull conservation — they are threatened too — and been glad to provide them with a safe haven. While brooding, the gull family was quiet, unless some movement from us below or from the sky above was taken to be a threat, and even then the response was a stiff but muted one, as if afraid to waken the egg too soon. Now the chick has hatched there is a great deal of activity; its own tremulous cheeping, and the parents' raucous screeching, calling across the valley to each other to bring food (as I imagine) over here, over here. And loud defensive calls and gestures at any potential threat. It's a bloody racket and hard to love when you're feeling sick.

This morning I stopped counting hairs after I reached 120 and saw that there were at least fifty more. Hair thinning is now an undeniable side effect. At least it doesn't show (how many hairs does the average head have?) but each one of them is incalculably more precious to me now.

Eleventh Letter

Dear Readers

I was given too-hefty doses, as a child, of a Westernised version of Eastern spiritualism that says we should be detached, that the wise man (it was always a man) is unaffected by the trials and sorrows, the highs and lows of this life, and fixes his mind in the Absolute (as we called God). That attempted detachment meant I took decades to grieve my mother's death when I was twelve, and it has made me wary of being too quick to leave the past behind.

So here I am wanting not to deny the trauma of Saturday's nausea, because I know how foolish it can be to pretend everything is all right and I am fully recovered, untouched even, by the pain. On the other hand, why hang on to it?

I want to learn, for myself and not through the clumsy diktats of others, how to embrace all that has been, is, and will be. Now, today: the sheer joy of hearing the rain on the window-canopy as I write, the cheeping of the gull chick and, because I'm feeling better, slightly more lovable raucous parents, the blue-grey sea that rises to the horizon and merges seamlessly with the white-grey sky, the green and granite-grey harbour arm pointing to France, the bright shingle beach, the glistening roofs of the Old Town, the chimney pots, my own sense of well-being. Rather than drag the pain of Saturday into this joy of now, I can simply acknowledge, with *gratitude*, that if it weren't for the cancer and its attendant grief, I might not have noticed or felt the deep joy of these quotidian movements of God's most glorious creation.

Tuesday, 11 June

Another exquisite moment. Waiting on Denby for our hack to start, I watch two horses in the adjacent field standing facing towards each other, but each with one cheek pressed gently to the cheek of the other, completely still: 'their hung heads patient as the horizons', as Ted Hughes puts it (thank you, I, for sending the poem).[8] 'They're keeping the flies off each other,' explains Rachel, 'but they are also just being with each other.'

I don't want to forget I have cancer. I want to have my mind concentrated by the ringing of my mortality bell. What will I make of this life that is left to me, 'whether it be short or long'?

Thursday, 13 June

A number of years ago I attended a first aid course. On the second morning, our teacher, Harry, a former fireman, took Resusi-Annie, the doll on which we practised our kisses of life and chest thumps, laid her out on a plastic sheet, and carefully poured a tin of chunky vegetable soup into her mouth. She had collapsed and vomited, Harry explained, and our task that morning was to resuscitate her. I was picked as the first in the group to do so. To me, the vegetable soup *was* vomit. It looked exactly like it. And I still think that going forward and putting my mouth to Resusi-Annie's revoltingly spattered mouth was among the braver things I have done in my life. (Like an idiot, concentrating too much just on the fact that I had to do this thing because she was dying and Harry had said I had to, I neglected to wipe the vomit soup away from her mouth, which would have made the kiss both more bearable and more effective. Everyone else after me did.)

I remember going towards Resusi-Annie as all the cells in my body seem to shrink and draw back from today's entrance to the tunnel of hard things: the early morning steroid dose, the blood tests, the first infusion, the sleepless night, the second infusion tomorrow, the nausea, the train journey, the nausea, the restless night and all day Saturday in Hastings just looking at the sea, the nausea . . .

I put one foot in front of the other and enter the tunnel of hard things. And as I enter, but only when I enter, I see again all the wonderful things in there too. First, the tunnel is bathed in love, in fact it is made of love. Second, it is populated by people showing profound, often unconscious, bravery. People walking towards their healing poison with their heads held high, not faltering. Their supporters by their sides, embodying equal measures of courage and pep. The groups clustering round patients cheering everyone up with their jollity, greeting each other as if this were a market place or a town square. Ebullient, strong, laughing, dignified. B, a wrinkled lady of considerable age, sits next to me in the blood test village, bright eyed, who has taken the trouble to apply mascara, lots of it. She shows me the size of her lymph node that has just started to grow, by pointing at one of her bright blue claw-like shellacked fingernails. She is naughty and alive, and deep in her eyes I see a calmness that as I write about it now brings tears to my own. They are tears of discipleship.

Sunday, 16 June

I have a horror of ending up satisfied with small things. Saturday is a day of small things, the day on which it is an achievement to drink three litres of water, take my drugs, eat a little bit, sleep, not vomit. Nothing else is required; nothing else is possible. On Saturday, my world is tiny. On Saturday, I cannot care for more than the very basic needs of my body. While our fragile, kicked-about Earth is disintegrating, and our fractious, factionalised people are pandering to populism, I am worried about my tiny self only.

I should not miss the divine in ordinary. Every minute movement of creation is a sign. Every minute movement is seen by God, loved by God, from God. 'Even the very hairs of your head are all numbered' (Matthew 10:30; Luke 12:7. Thank you, E).

Incarnate love. Our interstices are full, rich with silence and strength and love.

The interstices of my Saturdays of small things are filled with Seán's tender, funny service, incarnate love given without stint and a great deal of laughter. What could be small about that?

And the sea. I look at the sea a lot. Another gift. Then I remember B in the Cancer Centre. And as I contemplate the interstices of my tunnel of hard things and my day of small things, the interstices grow and grow until they are enormous, vastly bigger than the things, embracing the things, holding them, being there before them and still being there after they have passed, which they do, and they have done because now it is Sunday and I am *all right*.

Twelfth Letter

Dear Readers

We decide to try the recently refurbished Fagin's restaurant on the corner of George Street and the High Street in Hastings. It has a fresh French bistro feel, with stripped back floorboards and bentwood chairs. I have lamb. Chewy. Then the elderly man at the table next to us is. I cannot believe this. Sick. Beautifully and swiftly dealt with by sympathetic staff; I don't think the other customers at the front of the restaurant have any notion of the incident. Even Seán has his back to their table. Only I, for whom vomit has become a theme, for whom a week off treatment means I can have a week off either having nausea or dreading having it, only I am witness to the vomit. I know the world doesn't revolve around me, but it is as though a special show has been created for me. One night only. When Claire's here. A man throwing up.
    Poor fellow.

Friday, 21 June

Oh the cruelty of the insomniac's night made worse by Dexamethasone. The long hours during which sleep eludes me, a sweetness that I know is there, just by me, but denied me. And then, finally, I drop off and at that PRECISE moment two loud men begin an argument outside my window, and I am wide awake again. It is 3.00am. I drink a herbal tisane called 'Sleep' that tastes revolting and makes no difference. I read *Self's Punishment*[9] (thank you, K), a German detective story (in translation) and struggle to follow the staccato-rendered plot

79

and complex names. I read Barton's *History of the Bible*[10] (thank you, G) and am instantly irritated by his concern to pacify the biblical literalists — though not, to be fair, pandering to them. I tell the rosary and it brings nothing, no comfort, no peace of mind, no sleep. I throw the beads down in fury and frustration. Religion is useless. Oh, I just feel like shit.

Religion is no comfort to me. It doesn't bring peace of mind or steadiness or answers or happiness. But maybe these are not its point.

I have such an active mind, ready to be engaged with a subject given half a chance, not good at disengaging. Or rather, when it is tired, it doesn't know what to do with itself. It is used to being centre stage, looking after things, taking responsibility. Doing that properly, like this writing, takes an effort and an energy that isn't always there. But when one's joy is in those activities which require an engaged and active mind, like writing, where does one find joy when the mind needs to rest? Other leisure activities which I love, like singing, do use a different register, but they don't usually bring quietude, not the sort that allows sleep, anyway. And I can't sing in the middle of the night. Or go horse riding. I think that everything I do I tend to throw myself into wholeheartedly and that means my energy is always wide awake. ('She's very lively,' said our matchmaking friend to Seán.)

Glenda my Pilates teacher talks about the importance of releasing muscles after an exercise. We are prone to stick with either moving or holding ourselves in readiness to move, not releasing and resting from movement. It is stressful to be always either on the alert (the warrior pose), or busy doing (fight or flight). We have to cultivate a habit of relaxation.

She also points out that there are many kinds of meditation, and one will be right for me for now.

I was initiated into mantra meditation at ten and it remains my cherished and regular refuge. I have a Sanskrit and an Aramaic mantra and I love and listen to both. You have your one little word, as the author of the *Cloud of Unknowing* puts it, and it is like a 'sharp dart of longing love' that pierces the cloud about God's glory, sometimes bringing an encounter in which there is perfect rest. A glorious beholding. But as Julian would observe, from God's point of view, beseeching and beholding are the same. I have learned not to demand of the meditation that result, or do it in order to have that inexpressibly beautiful, divine feeling. And it isn't a sleep aid, because it requires a concentrated, focused attention that is by its nature wakeful.

The same goes for the rosary, another meditation.

I have also been meditating in a healing kind of way, entering imaginatively my body and especially the centre of my bones where the marrow is, imagining the cell-making that is going on there and good cells being made; then imagining them travelling through the porous bone itself to the blood, and my blood flowing around my body as a healing movement, full of love, countering the myeloma with love not war.

And I practise Ignatian meditation, which is both sensory and imaginative, deeply connecting with a scriptural text.

So plenty to choose from, but none of them is any use when I want to sleep.

Now: I simply listen to my breath. In and out, gently, sleep slowly creeping, seeping, towards me.

Saturday, 22 June

I have it on the excellent authority of Judith my hairdresser that it is safe to lose up to 200 hairs a day, providing they don't all fall out of the same place on one's head. At most I'm losing 200 hairs from all over my head when I wash it, which happens every other day. I continue to look entirely normal. At the moment. But writing about it has generated moving and practical responses from those of you who have gone through this fiendish test of one's peace of mind. I am inspired by your poem, A: 'Let others recognise and see a new shape', but the unhaired shape that is revealed has always been there. In as much as we are our bodies, we are our hair too, so I wouldn't say it is necessarily the case that 'the real me' would be revealed if I lost my hair; but it works brilliantly as a metaphor: all that I cover myself with has been taken from me. I am now much more aware of and sympathetic to men's mid-life hair loss than I was. If you feel even remotely as we do about your hair, and why wouldn't you, it must be traumatic. And unlike chemotherapy hair loss, yours doesn't come back. When I dress in the morning, I also dress my hair. Losing my hair, if I have to, will be a bit like losing my clothes. Naked I will stand before you: vulnerable and revealed; no secrets covered up.

One of the most moving crucifixes I have ever had the privilege to contemplate is in the oratory of the Church of San Spirito in Florence, on the unfashionable side of the Arno. It is an early piece by Michelangelo, quite small, carved in wood. The Christ is naked. His body is painfully young, almost adolescent, utterly revealed and unprotected. When we were last in Florence it was the first thing we saw, before we crossed the river to more familiar beauties. We stood transfixed for a long time. We wept. We left the church, then went back in again, drawn irresistibly to this figure that showed itself to us so completely. We wept again. I could have returned to London that evening, already entirely satisfied.

Perhaps I really am a Christian after all. I find this unprotected revealing, this allowing, this suffering to be done unto, of the crucifixion, the necessary passage to resurrection, the most powerful truth it is possible to be made known in this beautiful, chaotic, suffering, endlessly confounding world. Revelation of what we actually, brokenly are, is almost unbearably beautiful, and it stops me in my tracks, as many of your responses have, the ones in which you write so truthfully of yourselves. And whatever the resurrection is, because we pass through the crucifixion to realise it, it includes the crucifixion. Perhaps that is what Julian means when she writes: 'sin is behovely', because for Julian 'sin' is known only by the pain it causes.

I resonate with Julian when she wishes to experience the pain of the Passion. I'm not writing here about some masochistic urge to be hurt, but rather the absolute revealing of the truth of myself, *in extremis*, nothing covered up. Her eighth revelation is of the last moments of Christ dying on the cross, and her encounter with him in this extreme state is so porous that her wish is granted and she does indeed suffer the pains of the crucifixion. It is a pain worse than anything she has experienced or could have imagined before. A voice counsels her to look away from the cross and transfer her gaze straight up to heaven, but she refuses, understanding that she is looking at heaven already in the bloody, disfigured face of the dying Christ, battered and destroyed by the world he revealed himself to without any protection.

I just know that this is true: we have to go through the pain, or call it fear, not over it or around it. Because resurrection is here, not elsewhere.

Thirteenth Letter

Dear Readers

Tuesday, 25 June

I'm watching the gull chick, recently born in the nest on Laetitia's roof opposite our house, stumble up and down the space around him: is he learning to walk before flying?

I have such a surge of well-being and energy in the final trot home of our ride today. Energy into the body, through the body, through every cell. Willing good health and strength. I don't feel I am entirely dependent upon the drugs keeping me alive, though I will die without them. I am bringing something myself too, something forceful and porous, humble and stubborn. It doesn't feel like a force that will prolong my life so much as one that wills life in general. Actually, it doesn't feel as though it's from me at all; rather I feel it as a gift in me.

I feel hungry for life, and I am countering the force of entropy thereby. I am still creating my niche. 'Niche creation' is a concept I discovered in recent evolutionary theory.[11] Evolution isn't just genetic, it's also environmental, as we interact with what is around us, it changing us and we changing it. Creatures create niches – their home, the company they keep – and these are passed down through generations, so much so that it is possible to tell a species is present even if the creature itself isn't present, by the sort of nest it has built and the presence of the habitat and ecosystem in which it will survive and thrive. Similarly humans. Think of the different sorts of humans all over the world and the different ways in which we have all made our nests and our communities. Seán's niche which is immensely cluttered; my niche which is very tidy and ordered, which Seán calls 'impersonal'. You create your niche through interacting with 'affordances', the things and people and concepts around you. By interacting with them, choosing them, making them into something that is part of you — this cup for drinking tea; this music you listen to or perform; this person who becomes a friend or a lover; this life lesson you learn — what seems to be an object other than you becomes part of your subjectivity, and you part of theirs of course.

Affordances and niche creation help explain how encounter becomes porous, how we are not hermetically sealed off individuals but constantly responding and changing in our interaction with what looks, to our Enlightenment minds, like a world that is only outside ourselves.

I think there is a connection between the hunger for life that counters entropy, and affordances and niche creation. The move outwards to connect with those people and things that are around us is a movement of life. As I walk into the Cancer Centre, bracing myself for the next infusion, despite everything in me wanting to turn away and give up, I look at those around me and draw strength from them, my connection with them helping my resolve. The Centre itself is a source of strength, built to give life, designed to help us all cope and even thrive. The birdsong in the lift. The artwork. The light. The Dimbleby Centre with its reflexology and ultra-nice people.

I looked up 'interstices' just now to check I had used the word correctly and found 'interosculate' nearby, which is a lovely discovery and quite a good word for the porous encounter.

I'm writing about love, am I not?

Wednesday, 26 June

Through fear of infection, I have brought air kissing to a new level. I raise my hands to either side of my head, palms open, like some sort of Renaissance dance posture, then my head juts forward and I say mwah mwah, and try to look all that I feel. I am a tactile person, I realise, indeed we all seem to be more tactile now, and holding back physically from a welcoming embrace feels awkward and cold. I think I will work on the ritual, turn it into something symbolic related to affordances and interosculation. And then bore my bewildered interosculatee, who just wants to say hello, by explaining myself for ten minutes.

However, ritual greetings with no physical contact have proved fruitless in protecting me against the common cold, which I now have. It started on Sunday. The pre-cancer Claire would have overridden her body's state and gone to your book launch, N, that night. No more overriding for me. Forced to move at the pace of my own body, I tell myself this: cancer is aligning my body, mind and spirit, and that's a good thing. It's about time, Claire.

Monday brings a sore throat and Tuesday brings snot. But no temperature so I will still have chemotherapy tomorrow.

Nor does the cold prevent my singing lesson with Patrick today: there is nothing wrong with my voice. The strength in me rises up again as I sing: strength not to live for ever, but for life itself. I sing Ralph Vaughan Williams' music and George Herbert's words:

> Come my Light, my Feast, my Strength:
> Such a Light as shows a feast;
> Such a Feast as mends in length;
> Such a Strength as makes his guest.[12]

I nearly break apart as I sing 'strength' — *this* is the strength that wells up in me from time to time. I manage not to cry, and in the last verse, which is higher, to begin with louder, then falling away to almost nothing, I feel my whole self is the song. Yes. It is love.

Thursday, 27 June

Outside mothercare a Chinese patient lies barefoot on the sofa waiting to be called. His family surround him and one of them is massaging him all over.

I notice for the first time how many mothers-as-carers there are in mothercare. Their brave faces. One mother is here with her daughter who can be no more than twenty. A mother's pain held at bay for the sake of the beloved, while her heart is breaking.

Despite my cold, my pulse is sixty and my blood pressure is 123 over something: I've never been this healthy.

Today I have an addition to my treatment: Zometa. Zometa is the trade name for zoledronic acid, a bisphosphonate, that is, a molecule that binds to calcium and is taken up into the bone, and stops the breaking down of bone that happens in myeloma. I don't have myeloma bone disease (yet) but a clinical trial showed that the length of remission and overall survival rate was improved in all patients who received Zometa, some of whom had myeloma bone disease and some of whom didn't. So we all receive Zometa now because it has an anti-myeloma effect as well as treating bone disease.

Thank you, my fellow myeloma sufferers who were the research subjects in that trial.

Zometa will be given to me once a month as a fifteen-minute infusion, for twenty-four months.

Twenty-four months. I realise all over again that I have cancer, that I am living with cancer, that as things stand, the best I can hope for is that the myeloma will go into remission for long enough for me to die of something else.

What would be a desirable alternative cause of death, I wonder? Suppose you could choose how you were to die, Dear Readers, how would that be? A comedian I met during my summer of doing stand-up told me that in his culture the only way to die was over the age of seventy, in your own bed, with your children and grandchildren and great-grandchildren all around you.

Danny Finkelstein told this joke: Solomon is on his death bed and his dutiful sons are with him. 'Abe,' he croaks, 'Abe, come here.' Abe leans forward and puts his ear to his father's lips. 'I can smell your mother's beautiful gefilte fish,' Solomon whispers. 'Tell her, it'll make a dying man happy if she gave me some to eat.' Abe leaves the room and returns a little later, empty handed. Solomon looks at him, his face alight with hope. 'She says you can't have any,' Abe tells him. 'She's saving them for the funeral.'

Friday, 28 June

I didn't sleep too badly: maybe five hours, which is good for a Dexamethasone night. But Thursday's immense ingestion of drugs – Dexamethasone, Omeprazole, Acyclovir, Domperidone, vitamin D3 on top of Zometa, Carfilzomib, Cyclophosphamide – is a lot to take, and I have a cold. I walk slowly, each step unwilling, along Newcomen Street to the Cancer Centre. As I enter, I think of the strength of George Herbert's 'The Call'. I physically put my shoulders back, I psychologically gird my loins. I connect with the Centre building, the other patients, and the staff and volunteers. I make myself ready to receive – gladly – today's infusions. I interosculate. I shall interosculate my drugs.

I cannot actually gird my loins, as it happens, as I am wearing a pair of those knickers that boast no Visible Panty Line, a selling point which simply means in practice that they have no elastic so that after one has worn and washed them a few times they don't stay up. Luckily I am wearing trousers, though they are baggy wide-legged ones, so I am in theory safe, but it's all very liberated as I make my way into the Centre and find a lavatory and make adjustments.

Saturday, 29 June

The gulls are screaming across the valley, a searing racket from the early hours and continuing all day. I would like to kill the chick on Laetitia's roof, and the one on ours. And every other gull in Hastings. I feel nauseous. Really nauseous: I come closer to actually throwing up than I have done hitherto. I have a cold. Why is it called that? I am *hot*. I am having hot flushes, the sweat running like water down my skin. Am I hot because the day is hot, or because I am having hot flushes, or because I have a temperature?

I don't want to take my temperature. I cannot abide the Conquest Hospital today, at thirty degrees. That windowless cupboard, 'deep-cleaned' with the bit of carrot on the table. That slippery plastic trolley. That bathroom.

I take my temperature. I cannot be irresponsible about this. It's 37.3 degrees, just 0.2 degrees below the danger zone. I think cool

thoughts, drink water, lie still, read the inspiring, mercifully distracting autobiography of Dame Steve Shirley,[13] thank you, N. And, in
your card with 'pep in your step' on the front, your memory, J, of
riding in the New Forest with A and me when we were schoolgirls,
when your horse sat down while you were still on it, makes me
laugh out loud. I take my temperature afterwards and it has come
right down. Temporal proximity does not equate to causality but
laughter does make you feel better. Wouldn't that be a grand clinical
trial? To discover whether laughter reduced your temperature. I bet
it does. And nature. Imagine a 'wilded' hospital. What a paradigm
shift: bugs are *welcome* here.

I cannot bear feeling ill. Or rather, I can bear it, but only because
I know that it will be over by tomorrow. I think: Suppose there
comes a time when *this* won't be over tomorrow, but is my new
normality? How will I bear it? I could not bear it. Life would not be
worth living.

But Steve Shirley had a profoundly autistic son who lived with far
worse than anything I am going through today, and she and her
husband lived with it too, until their son died in his thirties.

Why would you keep on living? That is not a rhetorical
question.

Sunday, 30 June

When I awaken, the gull screaming is further away and quieter, or
perhaps it is just that I have recovered and it no longer intrudes. I am
myself again. I think: every week I have an Easter Saturday and an Easter
Sunday, a day of feeling like death and a morning of resurrection.

Fourteenth Letter

Dear Readers

The reason I don't go to big evangelical services is not because I don't like them or agree with them but because, if I did, I would break apart. Like a dam bursting. And I can't do that in public, can I? Fr Eamonn's sermon yesterday nearly had the same effect. 'Do you love me more than these?' asks Christ of Peter (John 21:15). Not: do you love me more than these other people do, but do you love me more than anything else in the world? Julian did. I don't know whether I do, I just know the effect the question had on me. It feels as though there is an enormous . . . love . . . waiting, but if I say yes to it I will . . . I will . . . not be able to cope.

I am being interosculated.

I am sweating. I tell my body, fondly, that I would sweat if I had all those drugs in me. I am consciously encouraging my body, telling it how well it's doing, imagining the blood being made in my bone marrow, and flowing out, being cleared of the myeloma cells through the drastic treatment.

Glenda, my Pilates teacher, says a bracing thing about my forearms, punctured and bruised by the cannulas they have received, that they are the frontline of my treatment. Courage, *mes braves* forearms! You will have to stay on the frontline: Grace has told me I can't have a port now because I might have a stem cell transplant later and it would be a source of infection.

Tuesday, 2 July

At the stables, sitting on a bench in the sunshine, in bliss, waiting to ride. The school, which is outdoors, is high up, so you can enjoy watching whatever is happening in the arena at the same time as glorying in the mellow Sussex countryside, and the sea sparkling in the distance.

As I bask, Grace phones with the results from the second cycle. I close my eyes, preparing myself to be disappointed. I cannot let these results determine my peace of mind. But they are good again: the kappa light chains, which had gone from 1,100 to fourteen after the first cycle, have stayed down. Stayed normal. And the paraproteins, which had gone down from eleven to six, are now at four. I am still responding well. Of course: I am so happy! And now Otis my horse is perfect, the sunshine is perfect, the landscape, in general and in the tiniest detail of this particular butterfly lightly landing on this leaf, this very leaf here, is perfect. My lovely friends at the stables rejoice with me, and at the presence of Sophie's newborn daughter, Rachel's granddaughter, who is here with her tiny perfect eyelids and toes and nose igniting little sparks of joy in us all.

Later I swim in the sea. It reminds me of eternity. And my own current physical limitations. I swim out to collect a floating plastic bag to put it out of harm's way and I am breathless and a bit panicky. I can't rush into spurts of activity as I have been used to. I have to move in the moment, relatively slowly. Not move to achieve, just move. I can't live that life where so many tasks are done on the way to other tasks: I'll just quickly clean this while the kettle's boiling; iron that while my bath's running; post the other on the way to the bus stop. Each of the little infill tasks has to become an action in its own right. It's much less exhausting and it does make me appreciate the beauty of ordinary things. And think about domesticity. For someone who has a job and fits household management around it, so many of those domestic tasks are slipped into the interstices between other seemingly more important things, and they become burdensome and stressful because they take time and I haven't really allowed time, don't feel I can afford to. Now all my interstices are becoming more important by the day.

Thursday, 4 July

I'm in the Cancer Centre. I watch a younger fat lady push an older fat lady in a wheelchair. Mel who runs The Wardrobe, a shop selling second-hand designer clothes and a great favourite in Hastings Old Town, told me about a friend of hers who, when her cancer finally confined her to a wheelchair, delighted in the fact that at last she could wear high heels without them hurting.

In mothercare receiving my infusion, I listen in to the conversation between the two ladies in chairs opposite me, one white Eastern European, the other Black African. They have teamed up to say the rosary together. I'm moved and say a Hail Mary as I swallow my oral chemotherapy tablets. Mary, mother, belongs in here.

Watching my fellow patients, I type this with one hand as the cannula for my infusion is close to my left elbow and moving my left arm sends the drip machine into bleep mode: 'the patient says to reflexologist are you married? your husband will never leave you. He must be brilliant if you do that to him all the time. And we are all laughing in our bay. Now i'm weeping. o god i love my fellow humans.'

M, you ask – thank you – why we can't respond to the realisation of our mortality with relaxation rather than intensity? What a great question. When I think about dying, I tense into warrior pose and feel spurred to action: fight or flight. But when it comes to it, neither of those responses will be any use at all; they'll only agitate me and make me rubbish and unhappy at dying.

Life will go on after death: I read a lovely story in Claire Tomalin's autobiography[14] – for which many thanks, R – of how, at the reception after her father's funeral, she had looked in on his great-grand-children who had been sent to his bedroom to play. They were, all four of them, jumping happily up and down on the same bed in which only a day earlier he had died.

Fifteenth Letter

Dear Readers

L'Arcelle, the mare I ride this morning, is delicate and sinuous but a lively ride; I hurt my middle muscles in the first slightly bouncy cancer [sic] as I get used to her and now I can't laugh or cough.

On my return to London I find an appointment letter from UCLH, University College London Hospital, waiting for me. This presages the start of the stem cell harvesting and possible transplant process. I haven't been given much of a gap between ending the four cycles of chemotherapy on 16 August and starting the next phase. But I would rather be getting on with things, especially things I ABSOLUTELY DREAD. I discover − my next shock − that I have to give myself the injections of growth hormones before the stem cell harvest, God help me. But you just get on with it, as I have seen my fellow cancer sufferers do, bravely and determinedly. You just do.

Wednesday, 10 July

JF takes me and Seán to supper at Tas in The Cut, and we sit discussing philosophy, spilled out on to the pavement in the warm night. JF is French and it feels very French. We discuss the feeling of familiarity we have towards famous figures that is, for obvious reasons, not reciprocated. I recall walking behind Jenni Murray into the auditorium at the Royal Court Theatre and, with as much familiarity as if she had been my sister, reaching up and tucking the sticking-out label back into her dress. Such an invasion — the nape of one's neck, for heaven's sake — but to her credit she didn't leap a foot in the air and scream blue murder. She turned and thanked me.

Thursday, 11 July

Today the self-check-in machine at the Cancer Centre rejects me because according to its newly programmed algorithm I am too early (but I've come for bloods, not chemotherapy, as I cannot explain to the machine). Patients arriving too early will clog up the waiting areas and create the wrong waiting-time statistics. We queue up to check in with a human being, overriding the programming glitch created by our anxiety not to be late.

Jared Diamond calls the need to be early 'constructive paranoia'.[15] You allow plenty of time for things to go wrong. Not being in a hurry changes everything, almost always for the better. Sodding machines.

Waiting for my blood tests I sit behind a man whose raised arm is inconveniently blocking the screen where our names appear, but he is gently stroking his bald head and I am touched. It is lovely and shiny and smooth, apart from some random small incisions that look as though someone has got at him with a small blunt instrument. It makes me think of those ancient skulls which show evidence of the person having died by having his head cleaved in. Evidence hidden by the layers of skin and hair. But what would cause this man's indentations? An over-enthusiastic gouger of a barber? I wonder if I have any dents in my scalp.

Ensconced in my purple chair: the couple opposite me are a man and a woman, the man in the chair, the woman at his side. The woman is reading the *Mirror*, whose front-page headline is 'Man with No Shame' over a picture of Boris Johnson. The man is reading the *Sun* whose front-page headline is: 'Intruder at Palace as Queen Slept'.

The lady to the left of the couple is the civil servant whom I've seen before. Or is she an author? Or a librarian? Clever, anyway. On the right is a slip of a young thing who looks both stoical and fierce even as she sleeps. She moves me.

An older, rough-cut man, wrinkled and hirsute, is to my immediate left, whose companion talks animatedly in Russian to him, making him laugh. She is young and her face is bright.

Then I discover that the clever lady is indeed a civil servant, but more importantly she, F, is also in the Cardamon trial, and a year ahead of me, so her knowledge of what happens, which she shares, is invaluable. She wasn't randomised to the stem cell transplant but to the second round of Carfilzomib, lucky lady. But she still lost her hair! It was the stem cell harvest chemotherapy, she tells me. She says that the clinicians said they had never seen that before so it shouldn't happen to me. Though she now sports a wonderful head of wavy, elegant grey hair and I think: that's not so bad. We talk and talk. There are some questions only other patients can answer.

Later, an hour of silence in a garden, thank you, J, for the suggestion, a still-consecrated space next to All Hallows Church in Copperfield Street, near the flat. My prayers are interrupted by the staff of the Church of England's Pension Board on a treasure hunt.

Friday, 12 July

Oh what an awful night! Awake, hot, tossing and turning, and quite badly nauseous. After talking to F I had started to feel such a fraud, such a lightweight in the scheme of cancers and cancer treatments . . . Well I'm not.

I am sick this morning.

My first time. Och, it wasn't too bad, more like (look away, squeamish ones) a liquid retch, and I think it was because I had some fruit last night: mango and cherries. There was nothing wrong with them but they were too rich and colourful. I'm having a cup of tea now and feel fragile but not nauseous anymore. Just the way anyone would feel who hadn't had much sleep.

Saturday, 13 July

On my nausea-induced sabbaths, as soon as I start to think 'What shall I do?', I feel queasy again. Is this like those alcohol-dependency

94

therapies or, God forgive us, those anti-homosexual therapies where you take a drug which makes you feel violently sick if you have or think about the thing you're supposed to be renouncing? I could think of my nausea days like this: curing me of my addiction to achievement.

Sunday, 14 July

Julian's ninth revelation. She has witnessed, and experienced in her own body, the pain of the dying Christ on the cross in the eighth revelation. Now she looks with all her might to see him dead, but she does not. She sees, instead, the same bloody, disfigured Christ transformed into bliss:

> And I looked after the departing with all my might and wende to have seen the body all dead, but I saw him not so. And right in the same time that methought, beseeming, the life might no longer last and the showing of the end behoved needs to be, suddenly, I beholding in the same cross, he changed his blissful cheer.

I wake up this morning, looking the same pallid mess I was yesterday, but I am merry. The world is the same and yet everything is different.
Sunday: resurrection day.

Sixteenth Letter

Dear Readers

On the ride this morning, after we cross the railway bridge and join the track that winds gently downhill, deeply bathed in nature, I am at that precise moment in bliss. The scene is beguiling: full of summer fecundity, beauty-burdened trees dappling the light, a hundred different shades of green and a million patterned shapes of leaves and butterflies and dust. It is like paused music, but it isn't this particular beauty that I am appreciating. It is . . . what? Beauty itself, and I believe I would, or could, feel this whatever the time of year, whatever the skies hold. I feel as though I am being appreciated, not the other way around.

I weep. Lucky for sunglasses and the fact that we all face one way as we ride.

Wednesday, 17 July

I have come to know the teachers and the tiny children from a local nursery who make their way so precariously along the ruined pavement outside my London flat each day, heading for the park. The teachers and I have bonded over trying to get something done about the pavement. The children have discovered what an echo is as they call into the hallway of my building. And they have made me a card to say get well soon.

Thursday, 18 July

Bouncy Cancer by Claire,
dedicated to J who noticed my telling typo last week
No chemo today, hurray hurray hurray
I'm going out to play, hurray hurray hurray
Oh no I need the loo, boo hoo boo hoo boo hoo
I have to catch my pee, tee hee tee hee tee hee.

Friday, 19 July

I stumble back to the flat, along Newcomen Street and through Little Dorrit Park, clutching Seán, tears and mascara running down my face. I have just had my regular, end-of-cycle meeting with the consultant, and hear, actually hear, what I have been told before but not heard. Yes, I may live for some time with myeloma, a cure may even be found before I die of it, or I may live long enough to die of something else. I have accepted living with it, as a chronic disease, and spoken too blithely, it seems to me now, of the importance of not thinking of it as an enemy to be fought, because it is in my blood and my blood is all through my body and I have to live with the disease. I have accepted this. But in my imagination, especially since the results have been so good, the myeloma will be a quiescent presence, to be checked upon from time to time by the lovely haematology team whom I will look forward to seeing.

What I have not imagined is repeated treatments. Today the consultant says that once I am through this first line of treatment, we will 'hope for two to three years of remission'. It can be as short a time as seven months before the myeloma reappears. She had one patient – just one – who lasted thirteen years in remission. 'We hope for two to three years.' One myeloma marker – in my case the kappa light chains – might be reduced to normal, but then another one might start replicating, and will need to be treated.

So now I contemplate another ten years of life not just living with myeloma but being repeatedly treated for it. No one had not said that. But the bright, 'new treatments are coming on stream all the time' response to myeloma's incurability had not, in my mind, translated until today into 'you will be repeatedly treated'. Having been through treatment once, and I haven't hit the hardest bit yet, how can I want it ever to be repeated?

I weep. Oh, Dear Readers, this is so hard. I had started to think I would be on my way back to normal during the eighteen-month maintenance chemotherapy, and properly back to normal once it had finished, only needing the odd visit to Guy's to check all is in abeyance.

I will never be back to normal.

Yes, yes, of course there are those who live for decades without needing further treatment, and of course I may be one of them. But it does me no good to believe I might be that lucky.

But nor does it do me any good to assume I will be back having some new poison within a year of finishing this first round of treatment.

It is limbo, endless limbo, and if I am not careful, endless dread of what may be to come, looking up constantly in fear at the sword of Damocles swinging above me, knowing now the sharpness of its blade and the cruelty of its cut.

Back at the flat and alone, Dear Readers, I ROAR.

Four times.

In that roar I feel all the strength of life. A full acceptance, a readiness to meet it, whatever it brings, with bright intelligence and wit and creativity and determination to make it beautiful.

But I also feel my helplessness. I cannot control what happens to me. Nor can I control what happens to you, my beloved fellow humans. Nor, forgive me, can I be what I think you want me to be. I mean, forgive me for thinking I know what you want. That you want me to be restored to the old, pre-cancer Claire. To Claire-without-cancer. That won't happen, and I think you know that perfectly well, better than I.

Between us, what will happen can be made tremendous. The strength in the roar is − tremendous. Unearthly.

Later, awake in the middle of the night, I ask God for help, as a child would. I need help and I ask for it. I ask for it now, I ask it of you, my Dear Readers, and I will accept it.

★   ★   ★

I have spent my life paddling upstream, forcing the pace, trying to change things, change myself, go against the flow. It's what young people do, I think, and quite rightly. But the river of life flows inexorably to the sea. If I accept the inevitable, I can dare to take my paddle out of the water and let the river flow turn my boat around to face downstream. Now instead of furiously paddling I can use the oar to make the downstream journey flow beautifully, skilfully. I can learn to shoot the rapids. I can navigate around obstacles, or choose to let them halt my journey for a while and enjoy the view, knowing that the flow will take me on again in due course. On, always on, forwards to the sea.

Seventeenth Letter

Dear Readers

Your messages, your attentive silence, your companionship. Oh, Dear Readers, you have helped me. I feel a deep strength that is not just my own, barely my own at all, more a strength that I join. It rises to meet what is to come, steadfastly. J, thank you for 'the communion of saints' and the comfort of that mysterious phrase which I see embodied in all of you. And for 'heirs through hope of thy everlasting kingdom', dear R. You feed my soul.

I swim. The bliss of dissolving into water that stretches all the way to the horizon. Seán sits reading on the beach in a lovely striped Edwardian swimsuit (not really) and is my lifeguard and my constant. I let the water take me where it will and check from time to time to see where I am in relation to him. I feel safe.

Thursday, 25 July

From our point of view, Julian's really important work, decades of it, all came after her near-death experience of her visions. Seán reminds me of this and I am energised and encouraged. Life after (this) treatment: will I flourish as Julian did?

If I have to have a stem cell transplant I shall think of the time in hospital as time in my anchorite's cell.

We don't have much information about Julian, and it is not actually possible to conclude that the author of the extant texts is the fourteenth-century Norwich anchoress called Julian whom we know existed from other sources, because the manuscripts are all much later.[16] But Benedicta Ward's plausible surmise about her life[17] is that she was born in 1343, was a householder with at least one child, but lost her family to the plague. She suffered a near-death illness herself in May 1373 at the crisis of which she experienced sixteen revelations. After that, for more than thirty years, she was an anchoress in a room next to the church of St Julian in Norwich from where she dispensed advice and in which she reflected on what she had seen, and wrote the wonderful text about her revelations. An anchorite, of which there were some fifty in Norwich at the time, was someone who undertook to remain in a room attached to a church living according to simple vows. The room would have a squint into the church through which she or he could participate in the mass; and a window to the outside world so people could come to seek and obtain advice. She might have a servant in an adjoining room and a garden. She was not to go to extremes: she was to eat and sleep properly, but she would remain in her room for the rest of her life. As I contemplate the rest of my life after the crisis of my diagnosis and first, disruptive round of treatment, I think of Julian.

From Chapter 22, the ninth revelation:

> Then said our good lord asking: Art thou well apayd that I suffered for thee? I said: ye, good lord, gramercy; ye, good lord, blessed moet thou be. Then said Jesu our good lord: if thou are apayd, I am apayd. It is a joy, a bliss, an endless lyking to me that ever I suffered passion for thee; and if I might suffer more, I would suffer more.

'Apayd' carries the sense of 'pleased' or 'satisfied', not a financial transaction.

You know, I can't hear what Julian is saying. I can't hear that Christ would suffer more for me if he could. I can't feel the love whose working this is. I rejoice in Julian's 'ye, good lord, gramercy' but I don't know it for my own.

This morning I take time over my hair. The baby shampoo I'm using makes it squeaky and tangled, and I tear it as I drag a comb through it impatiently just as I used to as a small girl. I don't want to lose more than I have to, so I return to the shower, apply conditioner, and rinse. Combing it out is easy after that. There is time to take time. It is important.

Today in mothercare I see a hairbrush abandoned in the lavatory cubicle; a poignant presence.

Friday, 26 July

A smell which I deduce is a dead mouse (one had got in from our communal bin area) pervades the flat. I could not deal with it last night and Seán will only be here later to help. I wake and the smell increases my nausea tenfold, so that I do end up quite gloriously vomiting, but since I have only had (quite a lot of) water, it is a nice clean vomit, pints of water leaping back up inside me like salmon returning upstream and out like a waterfall into the lavatory bowl, relieving me.

There is no dead mouse, Seán assures me, having searched. The smell has gone by the time he arrives.

The hairbrush is still in the lavatory cubicle upon today's visit, but now, carefully placed next to it, there is a vomit bowl covered by a napkin. I avert my eyes. I'm not feeling well. No poignancy anymore, just nausea. And I am not helped, though my sympathy is raised sky-high, by a poor lady also receiving chemotherapy whose skin is everywhere horribly damaged, by radiation burns, possibly, or a rash. She is in good spirits. I am in awe even though my fragile stomach means I cannot look at her.

Saturday, 27 July

I am in my physically induced sabbath. Lovely drenching rain brings quietude — even the gulls are quiet — and the fishing boats are out. We count ten of them. I feel as though we are in a ship in Sunbeam House, with the view of the sea stretching to the horizon.

I watch the sea and I think of the Irish monks of Skellig Michael. They were inspired by the desert fathers like St Anthony, who left the metropolis to find peace and unmediated prayer in the Egyptian desert in the early centuries of Christianity. For the Irish monks, the sea was their desert, and they set sail westwards from Ireland with no prior knowledge of their destination, just as they imagined Anthony had set out into the desert not knowing what he would find. The next land mass is America, but eight miles from the Dingle coast, rising out of the sea, there are two small rocky islands, just two, the Skelligs, and on one the monks built their home; 600 stone steps fashioned as they climbed, up to the flat top of the rock where they built individual stone beehive huts and a communal chapel. They lived off fish, puffin eggs and the little they could grow from the guano that formed a kind of soil on the otherwise bare rock.

You cannot see the Skelligs from the coast. The monks would only find their new world once they had let go of their known world, and that's what I feel I'm being asked to do now, myself. As long as I hang on to who and what I was before the cancer diagnosis I will not be able to discover its creative promise which I truly believe is there, waiting to be realised.

Let go of the old, Claire!

Sunday, 28 July

I read, in Peter Reason's *In Search of Grace*,[18] of the 'post-heroic jour-ney', which, unlike the classic hero's journey, involves no physical departure, no great conquests or trials, but rather arises when the hero is undone by some sort of downfall: something challenges her and turns her world upside down. She is forced to discover what she is when everything is taken from her. She has to stay still.

Monday, 29 July

In church for an hour of blessed silence. Right at the end of the hour the question rises in my heart, all unbidden: 'Art thou well apayd?' and I hear Julian's reply, 'yea, lord, gramercy, blessed moet thou be'. It isn't my reply. I have no reply.

The question repeats itself. 'Art thou well apayd?'

And again: 'Art thou well apayd?'

I check the glossary of the text I have brought with me — which I have not done before — to make sure I understand what 'apayd' meant. Yes. 'Pleased, satisfied'.

Why, oh why, on Earth should Jesus or anyone, anyone at all, be so concerned to 'apay' me? But my tears silence my unbelieving heart.

Eighteenth Letter

Dear Readers

The ride on Denby is bliss, again. Because my back had gone into spasm from a too-eager leap into 'the shortest canter in the world' last week, I am much more attentive to tuning into his pace as he makes the transition from trot to canter this week. He is a solid fellow, and if I am not in tune with him, my behind bashes on the saddle with each leap forward of his stride. Today I find his measure and really enjoy the connected strength of a more mellifluous run. That and glorious nature. Glorious, glorious nature.

Before my diagnosis, when I thought I would live for ever, I nevertheless felt and acted as though the service to which I was called would not wait for me. I had to hurry into and through the tasks and responsibilities of my life, climbing fast and furiously, in order to reach this summit, then on to the next summit, and the next.

Missing the point. Not enjoying the journey. Not stopping to look at the view. Still, it was exhilarating. And it seems paradoxical that even as I hear my mortality bell ringing, I feel a call to slow down rather than cram everything in. Is this your 'relaxed' response to death, M?

Perhaps what I am feeling now, or wanting to feel, is a life lived at the pace of nature. Recognising due season, timeliness, unhurried Earth turning and sun rising. Death and rebirth, rotting and renewal, the force of life and the stillness of death.

That force of life encourages me to face down my fear of the stem cell transplant by addressing one of its biggest horrors: hair loss. I decide I will try on a wig.

Thursday, 1 August

I wake up depressed. My whole body feels literally fed up with the infusions and swallowings of so many chemicals. Just two more weeks of infusions to go, and then a break of sorts, I tell myself. To the kitchen for my 40mg of steroids. Urgh. I eat walnuts as I forgot to buy a banana. 6.00am is a bit early for walnuts. Two pints of water. Back to bed with a cup of tea. I don't know if I can face going into the wig shop.

Well. I arrive at the Cancer Centre for my morning bloods, and lo, there is a lady with a kind face sitting at a table with a heap of brightly coloured scarves, giving lessons in how to tie them on your head for when you go bald. As soon as I have checked in I sit down and ask for a lesson. I choose a lime green scarf and practise tying it on my head in different styles. I am clumsy but with Jenny's help I manage two shapes.

I am called for my bloods but, encouraged by Jenny, once I am free again I go into the wig shop and meet two beautiful young women who explain the system. I will receive a voucher for £250 to pay for an acrylic wig; or the money can be put towards a real-hair wig. Real-hair wigs look real; acrylic wigs look false. Acrylic wigs are easy to care for, but they can't be dyed or blow dried, whereas real-hair wigs can be treated like real hair, and last for longer. Real-hair wigs are advised if one needs a wig long term, but if I do need a wig it should be short term only, so I look at the acrylic wigs. False, yes, but stylish. They don't look all that fake.

The wig ladies are sure they can match my hair colour with the acrylic wigs, and they can style a wig to make it the same shape as my hair now. They can also provide 'top up' hair pieces if I just lose clumps of hair (oh God).

Rather like preparing for a no-deal Brexit (or, frankly, Brexit), I now have information to meet my personal worst case, which is being randomised to the stem cell transplant and losing all my hair. I can wear beautiful scarves and play with colour; and I can have a stop-gap wig.

The headscarf-tying workshop table has not been there before. I feel, when I see it, that the universe has somehow risen to meet me halfway, on the very day that I need help to face down one of my fears.

Saturday, 3 August

As the nausea abates I feel resilience return: 'afresh, afresh, afresh', as Philip Larkin writes[19] (thank you, C). And as Seán has said, with great confidence: You will make the best of what befalls you. You will make it work for you. Today, I believe that. I pray for the steady strength that is needed, the courage to set sail from my known shores but quietly, blown gently by the life force that tends against decay. Today I believe even better things can come of a life lived at the pace of nature than one lived too fast and too thoughtlessly.

Resilience means not leaping into tough things too enthusiastically since one is in it for the long haul. Resilience means not trying to be too efficient. You have to pace it, breathe deeply, take your time, allow plenty of elastic, learn to say no as well as yes. Not wasting valuable energy wishing you didn't have cancer but accepting all the good it has made possible.

George Herbert writes: 'Affliction shall advance the flight in me'.[20]

Sunday, 4 August

My difficulty in accepting that anyone should care if I was 'apayd' is addressed, somewhat, in the next part of Julian's ninth revelation in Chapter 23.

> . . . Christ said: If thou are well apaid, I am well apaid, as if he had said, it is joy and liking enough to me, and I ask not else of thee of my travail but that I might apaye thee.
>
> And in this he brought to my mind the property of a glad giver. Ever a glad giver taketh but little heed at the thing that he giveth,

but all his desire and all his intent is to please him and solace him to whom he giveth it. And if the receiver take the gift gladly and thankfully, then the courteous giver setteth at nought all his cost and all his travail, for joy and delight that he hath, for he hath pleased and solaced him that he loveth. Plenteously and fully was this showed.

I have thought that giving should require no acknowledgement on the part of the recipient. But here's Jesus wanting to know if Julian is well apaid. It is her assurance that she is indeed well apaid – 'yea, lord, gramercy, blessed moet thou be!' – that makes him then not count the cost.

Needy Jesus.

Today in his sermon Fr Eamonn talks about acknowledging the presence of Christ; this is what he directs us to in the meditation he always includes in his homilies, but he also says, 'there's nothing you need to do, Christ is already present'. The exchange, of Christ's presence and love and my reception of him, isn't transactional, surely? The love is unconditional, not in the least dependent upon my willingness or ability to receive it. But the implication in the Julian passage is that Christ's pain is only set at nought when he is assured of my pleasure and solace.

Now look, Jesus. I am undyingly grateful for this exquisite world you have wrought. Not just its beauty, geometry, majesty and unbounding greenness. Also its mad, fierce anger and terror, ugliness and malice, unfairness and desperate sadness.

Aah. I feel in myself now the fronds of loving life unfurl like young ferns even in the midst of pain and fear. And I am grateful again. Yea, lord, gramercy.

Is this (a taste of) salvation, Jesus? Is this what you died for? Is this you, resurrected? Is this what you *mean*?

Later in the day, we walk through Ecclesbourne Glen, on the East Hill out of Hastings Old Town. A gentle woodland walk, ancient trees calmly feeding my soul; the pace and green and softness entering my receptive self and settling me. I am utterly served. Yea, lord, gramercy.

Nineteenth Letter

Dear Readers

Tuesday, 6 August

My ride is mellifluous on the long-backed, sinuous L'Arcelle. Sophie leads us, back on her horse a matter of weeks after lengthy, painful childbirth (three days of labour, stitches, the sort of childbirth mothers understatingly and magnificently describe to each other as 'a difficult one'). I feel life in me quickening, echoing Sophie's energetic reconnection with her horse and the landscape she loves.

Elizabeth Gilbert (of *Eat, Pray, Love* fame) lost her lover last year, and found her way through the grief and back to life by writing. She talks about being a willing student of grief, that grief itself moves you through the landscape of grief. And she says that she is willing to feel whatever she has to feel, however painful, because if she is no longer able to feel, depression will follow. She is like Julian, who in her eighth revelation experiences, by her own request, the pain of Christ's crucifixion in her own body, and knows it for the worst pain there is. She writes: 'I thought: Is any pain in hell like this? And I was answered in my reason: Hell is another pain, for there is despair.'

Thursday, 8 August

Needy Jesus . . . Yes we can give and not require a grateful response, because the point of the giving is not the gratitude of the recipient but the act of generosity itself. But for the recipient . . . Well a gift does have to be received, doesn't it? You have to say 'yes' to it. If you receive it, it can save you, as nature is without a shadow of a doubt saving me. So is water. And your unfailing kindness, Dear Readers. AND chemotherapy, which I have to receive, not reject. So yes, Jesus is right to be needy.

All these saving gifts are acts of love and in Christian theology they are manifestations of the resurrected Christ. So — bloody hell — I *can* say 'Jesus saves me'. Very quietly.

And now I reflect that my grateful, porous reception of these gifts of love has arisen from my knowledge of my need. Deep knowledge of my need, but not knowledge I gained from asking: it has been visited upon me.

Julian's tenth revelation is of being led into Jesus' side, through the wound that was made at his crucifixion. Inside, she sees his cloven heart. The encounter between her and Christ is taken graphically to a new depth: this is not face to face, this is entering into Christ:

> With a good cheer our good lord looked into his side and beheld with joy, and with his sweet looking he led forth the understanding of his creature by the same wound in to his side within; and there he showed a fair and delectable place, and large enough for all mankind that shall be saved and rest in peace and in love . . . And with this our good lord said well blessedfully, Lord how I love thee; as if he had said, my darling . . . see thine own brother, thy saviour.

'My darling.' Irresistible.

In the blood queue at the Cancer Centre:

> wrinkly shrunken old man in a Stetson and too-large denim
>   waistcoat, skinny legs in chinos and boating shoes: he has
>   dignity though you might have found his clothes ridiculous
> bald old man in cardigan next to his wife, probably, who has the
>   tan of foreign holidays and looks healthy but she has a stick
>   and I wonder who is the cancer patient
> little lady in big spectacles clutching her big gold bag and peep-
>   ing at the world over the top of it
> tall thin lady with beautifully cut white hair

fat lady in blue turquoise dress and white cardigan peering at her
   phone
wispy-haired lady with a stringy neck and a kind, patient,
   anxious face just sitting.

The table where I learned to tie a headscarf last week has colouring
books and felt tips and crayons on it today. I notice it as I come in.
Has there been an activity there every time? I simply haven't seen it
before. As I leave, I see an older man in a suit, who looks as though
he was once a professional accountant or something like that, still
wearing a tie though he's old and ill, sitting alone, colouring in. That
makes me cry.

When I come back later for my chemotherapy infusion, I see one
lady who has what we think of as the typical cancer look: she is
shrunken, bald, that ancient heartbreaking patience in her eyes, slow
movements . . . But she is the exception here in this centre of excellence for cancer, full of people with cancer. Most of us look like
everyone else, and the only way you'd know we were the ones with
cancer is that we aren't wearing staff passes. This, I realise, is not
what I saw when I first came here. Then, all I seemed to see were
shrunken, balding, shuffling cancer patients.

How perception shifts.

Opposite me today is a handsome young white man reading the
Sun, whose headline runs: 'Micro Pigs on the Moon'. The young
man is being rude to his companion about 'Europeans'. I wish he
wasn't so handsome.

Things you might hear both at a funeral and in the bedroom, from
an old episode of *I'm Sorry I Haven't a Clue*:

> I didn't expect so many of you to come.
> Would you please rise?
> Lovely spread.
> What do you mean, clapping at the end's inappropriate?
> The vicar gave her a lovely service.
> At least it was quick.
> This is what your mum would have wanted.

Well, that went as well as could be expected.

Can I just start by saying how nice it is to see so many of you here?

This is harder than I expected.

It was the second stroke that did it.

Nice hat.

What's she doing here?[21]

I go to Redcross Gardens again for my hour of contemplation and am granted an hour's peace. I pray for some of you. How do I do it? I take each of you in turn into my mind-heart and feel you there, like Jesus receiving Julian through the wound in his side. When I have really settled with your presence, I imagine huge wing-like arms held out ready to receive you. As gently as I can, I place you in those embracing arms.

Friday, 9 August

Another bad night. But I think of the rivulets of perspiration as my wondrously wrought body sweating out toxins and cannot be sorry that it happens. I move slowly today, and the cannula goes in first time, and the infusion is soon over, and the train is on time, and I put on my noise-cancelling headphones, rejoicing in their beautiful red-gold colour, and listen to *Our Mutual Friend* read by Simon Vance as I watch the Kent and Sussex green hills and woodland flash past, and before I know it we are safely in Sunbeam House and I can stretch out on my bed and look at the sea, and rest.

Saturday, 10 August

And today, although I don't have any energy or appetite, I don't feel sick. Some waves of nausea like a swelling sea with waves not breaking, that is all. I have organic cornflakes with milk for breakfast, a slice of white toast and honey with a cup of tea for lunch, but by supper time I am feeling hungrier and eat new potatoes with butter and pepper, some celery heart and a hard-boiled egg. I struggle to drink all my water ration, but I manage, helped by the addition of ginger recommended by F.

Today is my sabbath, and not one in which I have felt ill all the time. But I have been cautious, and not gone anywhere or done anything strenuous: a jigsaw puzzle while listening to Radio 4 and more of *Our Mutual Friend*, looking at the rumbustious sea whipped by a high wind and the lashing rain rattling the loose Georgian window frames. Loving Seán.

I love Radio 4. Once when there was a threat that it would be taken off long wave, a protest march took place along the Strand in London. The chant?

> What do we want?
> *Radio Four*
> Where do we want it?
> *On long wave.*
> What do we say?
> *Please.*

I was going to ask you to rejoice with me, Dear Readers, as I have now received my last infusion until I'm randomised to transplant or consolidation chemotherapy, which by my calculation won't be until 31 October. Brexit Day. My birthday. (I shall wear black.)

But. Last infusion? The monthly Zometa infusions carry on; there'll be another bone marrow biopsy and heaven knows what other tests to see how I've responded to the induction chemotherapy, then the stem cell harvest which involves more chemotherapy . . . there is no end. So best not to think of ends. Of any ends. Moments of rejoicing for what is now.

Sunday, 11 August

The sea calls and we head there for a swim. En route we visit Lois, whose myeloma is more advanced than mine. She is an inspiration and her hope for more treatments, of which she has only two left available to her, puts my grizzling at my own meagre side effects to shame. She is an inspiration because she is learning to accept death, and she teaches me. I hope I will have your spirit, Lois, when I am where you are.

★   ★   ★

I am reading Mary Colwell's *Curlew Moon* and Helen Macdonald's *H is for Hawk*.[22] I worry about the speeded-up world where technology forces a pace too fast for nature. The symbiosis between humanity and ecosystems has been disrupted. Seán tells a story from his childhood summers in Ireland in the 1950s. A small boy, he would go into the fields near his grandparents' cottage in Kerry during harvest. The men would be scything, and Seán would wait to catch field mice as they leapt out of the way of the steadily swishing long blades. At noon the Angelus bell would ring from the church a quarter of a mile up the hill in Knockanure village. Seán's grandfather, the overseer, would doff his cap and call out: 'The angel of the Lord declared unto Mary', and all the workers would doff their caps, sink to their knees in the fields where they were, and repeat the responses and the Hail Mary of the Angelus:

> Hail Mary, full of grace,
> the Lord is with thee;
> blessed art thou among women
> and blessed is the fruit of thy womb, Jesus.
> Holy Mary, mother of God,
> pray for us sinners now
> and at the hour of our death. Amen.

A decade later, the combine harvester arrived. The field became too dangerous for a small boy. The mice were minced in the fast-whirring blades. The Angelus bell could no longer be heard. I think: the machine racket has silenced humanity's humility and nature is suffering.

Twentieth Letter

Dear Readers

Tuesday, 13 August

I ride lovely, lithe and, as it turns out, extremely lively Nutkin. She is the mare I rode the week immediately following my diagnosis and so an arc is created by our joining again now, after my last induction chemotherapy infusion. I feel my thanks into her through my body for holding me then and holding me now, when I know I am much stronger and calmer and accepting about having cancer. Jess comes over with a young helper to check my girth and stirrups, and says to her: 'Nutkin is balanced, and so is Claire'. Yes. Rebalanced and in no small part because of these life-giving rides, which didn't throw me when I was thrown by the diagnosis.

Wednesday, 14 August

Thank you, H, for sending *The Idler* by Elizabeth Jennings, encouraging a new kind of letting-go attitude in me:

> Watch how a landscape kindest is to idlers
> Helping their shiftlessness grow to new powers,
> Composing stillness round their careless will.[23]

Friday, 16 August

In for the Zometa infusion which although not chemotherapy still takes place in mothercare. The childlike lady who is covered in radiotherapy burns or some other ghastly rash, whom I saw last week, is in a chair opposite, and because I am not feeling nauseous today I do not have to blank her. She has a truly sweet face. Big spectacles and wide-open eyes behind them. Her little hands are curled up painfully like claws. But she sits solving crossword clues with her mother, thanks the nurse for the cannula when it is in, despite the intense pain of insertion into her scaly-sore skin, and looks brightly on the world. She is not sorrowful, not now.

Next to her an older man is having oxygen as well as chemotherapy. I hear him say that at home he is on oxygen all the time apart from mealtimes. He sits quietly and breathes carefully.

I am very lucky. In an unlucky kind of a way, says Seán.

Twenty-first Letter

Dear Readers

On Holiday in York

Prospero's closing speech, heard today at a production of *The Tempest*, moves me greatly:

> Gentle breath of yours my sails
> Must fill, or else my project fails,
> Which was to please. Now I want
> Spirits to enforce, art to enchant,
> And my ending is despair,
> Unless I be relieved by prayer,
> Which pierces so that it assaults
> Mercy itself and frees all faults.
> As you from crimes would pardoned be,
> Let your indulgence set me free.

The utter loss of his power resonates, and his consequent utter dependence on the rest of humanity. I am not a hermetically sealed individual. I am all that I am because you are. How I feel this now, writing to you, Dear Readers.

At the Community of the Resurrection, Mirfield

I come to the monastery for silence, retreat, to join the Brethren for their cycle of prayer and to seek their guidance, to be left alone to reflect, pacing meditations in the grounds, stillness in the church; and to prepare for the coming months.

I make my confession.

Imagine: you have done all sorts of things you are sorry for, but you can't say sorry directly, either because what you have done is too pervasive, such as collusion in actions that damage the planet or communities on the other side of the world; or because the hurt is to yourself; or because it would only increase the hurt to say sorry. (A friend's seventeen-year-long relationship came horribly to an end when her partner confessed to seeing another woman. He then tried to tell her about all the other women with whom he had had affairs during their relationship, wanting to make a clean breast of his errancy. His wish to cleanse his soul utterly devastated my friend. He needed to take his sorry self to a priest or a therapist, not burden the one he had betrayed with his need to repent.)

This is what I do to prepare for confession. I spend some time, some considerable time, looking through the months since my last confession, and I identify as honestly as I can what I have done or said or thought which I feel sorry for. It has been eight months, and I am seeing myself more clearly than before, so the list is long:

Pushing away kindness because I have a low opinion of the form it takes; or it is so clumsy as to be hurtful.

Being impatient of help because it doesn't come at the time or in the way I want it to.

Being stupidly demanding of myself; expecting to be the same person functioning at the same high octane, speedy pitch, while reeling from the cancer diagnosis; the prognosis; the tests; the news of treatment regimes; fears about chemotherapy; the treatment itself.

Behaving strangely and tensely towards others, upsetting and worrying them.

Being harsh in telling the news that I have cancer, forgetting what a scary word it is, and how I become someone scary as a result.

Hanging on to responsibilities and preventing my
   colleagues from getting on with work by not letting go
   of it myself.

Failing to express or act on my needs, for example self-protec-
   tion from infection, and ending up behaving ungraciously out
   of fear, instead of graciously out of need.

Taking Seán for granted: every nanosecond I have done this.

Thinking I know better.

Worrying away at who I think I should be and what I should be
   doing, instead of hearing and responding to what God is calling me to be.

Not, simply, putting God first, but endlessly worrying about me.

Not acknowledging the myriad ways in which God shows God's
   love for me.

At this point in my preparation for confession, having dug through
the layers of things I feel bad about, I hit anger. At last. Now these
thoughts rise to the surface: I have tried so hard in my life to do the
right things and think the right thoughts and believe the right beliefs,
and what happens? I get cancer. That is my reward. I am angry and
I've only now felt it, after three quiet days at the monastery, and
being given the chance to look deep into my soul to prepare for
confession.
   I'm blazing with fury.
   The list continues:

Not understanding or believing the weakness of Christ.

Wanting recognition for all my efforts in my work and service
   when all I got was this lousy cancer.

I say all this to my confessor, ending in floods of tears as I speak about my anger, and find it impossible to say that I am truly sorry. I'm not, I'm angry. It's such a relief to feel it and to say so.

My confessor suggests, mildly, that I stop being so hard upon myself and gives me the hymn 'Love Divine all Loves Excelling' to read as my penance. An exquisite hymn which I sing through a few times and cry a lot. I acknowledge with relief that my own gargantuan, ultimately puny, efforts have ended in failure. I can't do this (whatever it is) myself. Which is what Prospero said, but maybe it takes a lifetime to realise it.

Lois has died. She had written this about her death:

> The idea of cold, of my body getting cold as death approaches fills me with fear. I want my lover to lie beside me and hold me tight. To whisper words of love and to keep me warm with his body, his words, his love.
>
> This would be the way to die. To drift off safe and warm in his love and with the wings of flight close by to carry me onwards.

I learn that Lois did indeed die in her husband's arms. Her breathing changed; he asked if he should call an ambulance; she said no, lie here with me in your arms. And there she died. Brave, brilliant Lois, I salute you.

In London

I have my first visit to UCLH. This is where the stem cell harvest will happen and where, if I am randomised to have it, the transplant. Yet more deeply impressive clinicians, another state-of-the-art cancer centre. And round the corner, the funny hotel-like place on Tottenham Court Road where you stay if you are having a transplant. We go and look: it is indeed just like a hotel, only all the guests are patients. Two badly dressed men sit in the lounge, talking.

III

Second Part of the Treatment

Twenty-second Letter

Dear Readers

Thank you, Dear Readers, for being here to write to as I lift the lid of my laptop and start tapping again at the keyboard. This is a long haul and I value your company so much. Thank you, J, for sending this poem by your friend which shows me where to look for strength in the everyday, to face my ongoing, gruelling every days.

> To open the stove door at dawn
> and find some embers still aglow
> within their comfy bed of ash
> and to build this morning's fire upon them
> and with focused breath
> to burst it into flame
>
> It's as if some kind old soul
> has been praying for me all night long
> watching over me
> keeping the faith
>
> To peg my shirt and underwear around the warming chimney
>   pipe
> and to put the kettle on
> to make my morning cup of tea

To clothe my nakedness
in the welcome warmth
of this relay race of grace

To sit by this window
and write this poem
whilst the sun
(from whom all light and fire and flame proceed)
rises gloriously through the morning clouds
to burst upon the sea
a path of such dazzling and inviting light

This
is the medicine
that daily
brings me back to life[1]

Tuesday, 10 September

I am deliciously back on a horse. Denby the mountain, hurray! Jess adjusts my stirrups and leans on him as we wait for the ride to start. He stands unmoving, our stable rock.

At the end of the summer there is a window of time when the farmer has cut his fields and hasn't yet ploughed and sown them with seed for the winter crop. When the fields are cut we can run across the middle of them. That time is now, and our ride is a wonderful, free, collective gallop across fields; we are like cowboys and maybe the horses feel it too, a herd again; none of the neat trotting and cantering in single file along the edges of the fields but out in open country, a familiar place looking utterly different, as you observe, H, and Denby coursing along, actually very safely and comfortably. Exhilaration in the rushing wind and the movement and the connect-edness of my body, his body, the air, the trees, the light, the open ground. And then as we quietly walk back, a long way because we have run a long way, we feel the stillness of summer drawing to a close under our eyes: hints of autumn in the odd fallen leaf already; a gentle bite of chilliness when a cloud crosses the sun; expectation in the air, not like spring, not lively, but with a soft melancholy, a welcome one. Now, feels nature, now is the time to prepare for rest, now my ebullience retreats, now I withdraw, settle, and soon I will sleep.

Thursday, 12 September

Lois' funeral was yesterday. She had written about her fear of the coldness of death and, oh, what a moment to catch my breath and weep as when the coffin arrived, the hearse led by a long thin man with a long grey beard and a long top hat − I want him for my funeral − we saw that it was covered in one of Lois' shawls and the simple sprig of wildflowers rested on a cushion. Keeping her warm.

When the curtains were drawn around the coffin as it was committed to the flames, we all, at Lois' request, applauded her and sent her on her way, clapped and cheered and shouted *brava*, and we all wrote prayers on pieces of paper and they went with her too.

And we mourned our loss. Why, at so many funerals, do the ones who have died insist they want a celebration and lots of laughter? The minute we are told this, we sob the more. We need to cry − the Lord knows I have learned this from my long, long grieving for my mother that did not begin at her death as it should have done but much later.

I am reminded of a story, told by the late Margot Jeffreys. At a conference in Jerusalem on national health services, the representative from Britain boasted of an NHS that cared for people from womb to tomb. The representative from Canada said: we do better, our health service looks after us from sperm to worm. The Israeli host capped their claims: our health service, he said, is the only one in the world that provides care from erection to resurrection.

Twenty-third Letter

Dear Readers

Tuesday, 17 September

Today I ride Wooster, a rare treat, a horse with a gorgeous temperament: calm and unflappable, a placid walker, a comfortable, easy trot, and a devil in him sometimes. He goes like a rocket in the canter and is hard to hold back. I love it. But the fields are all ploughed now so our glorious free runs across them are at an end for another year. And some of the fields have been ploughed right to their perimeters, so we can't even go around them. We will slowly remake the paths during our rides over the coming weeks, but it's a blow.

In her book *Late Fragments*,[2] Kate Gross writes of finding one's *cantus firmus*. This is a term in music meaning the melody which is the basis for a polyphonic composition, but Kate uses it to mean one's soul around which the harmony of others moves. The polyphony of others expands and contracts the sound of a life, revealing its beauty with glorious settings, and sometimes hiding it, with refrains that repeat themselves, for example our characteristics, our habits, and then with new expressions, reaching skywards or Earthwards, or inwards to the centre of the stave, pulling the soul into new shapes, then restoring it, settling, down, down, to a single note, then silence. Perhaps it takes a lifetime, short or long, to hear a *cantus firmus*. It's good to listen for it, amid the myriad harmonies and cacophonies of a life. It's another, more poetic way of thinking about niche creation. And interosculation.

I feel my *cantus firmus* glory when I am on a horse, and the horse and the countryside and I make polyphony. I feel certain that the harmonies and also the cacophonies that weave themselves around my *cantus firmus* change it. The melody of my soul responds to the company it keeps.

You send me this from Martha Nussbaum, dear G, which speaks of a related kind of interosculation:

> To be a good human being is to have a kind of openness to the world, an ability to trust uncertain things beyond your own control that can lead you to be shattered in very extreme circumstances. In circumstances for which you are not yourself to blame. And I think that says something very important about the condition of the ethical life, that it is based on a trust in the uncertain, a willingness to be exposed, that we're more and more like a plant than a jewel — something rather fragile, but whose very particular beauty is inseparable from that fragility.[3]

Ah yes, that is it. More like a plant than a jewel.

Wednesday, 18 September

I cycle to UCLH for my pre-harvest blood tests, relishing my route. I cycle all the way along quiet, evolving Webber Street, where low warehouses are being turned into charming apartments, with the Old Vic standing staunch and jaunty at the far end. Waterloo Bridge, an ugly (I think) structure itself, is the best bridge for crossing the Thames in central London, because it spans the river at the top of its most horse-shoe point. You have, looking from left to right, glorious views of the grandiose neo-Gothic Houses of Parliament with the modestly 'hunched shoulders' (as G.K. Chesterton called them) of Westminster Abbey behind; the river-facing hotels and clubs along the Strand, stately Somerset House and the barbaric post-war building of King's College; the elegant gardens and filigree stonework of the Temple Inns of Court, St Bride's wedding cake spire, the dome with its blindfolded statue of Justice surmounting the Old Bailey (which you can't actually see but it is there), the massive dome of St Paul's (which, since I saw Wren's model, I have thought to be a bit on the small side, proportionally), and the sprouting show-off skyscrapers in ever more fantastical shapes of the City, with Tower Bridge, the Tower of London and HMS Belfast just around the bend. A panorama to distract from safe cycling. Magnificent. Achieving the north side of the river, I cycle across the Strand and up Wellington Street, past the civilised edifice of the Royal Opera House, up Drury Lane to Long Acre, diving into Endell Street, which was Hogarth's Gin Lane. Although dead-smart Covent Garden now, it still maintains a seedy air. I turn right on a charming one-way detour into Betterton Street where the Poetry Society lurks, left and back on to Drury Lane again, across New Oxford Street and up Museum Street to the great British Museum herself; right around that grand and portly building, up Montague Street to Russell Square, Montague Place and finally Malet Street. I dock my bicycle here, between the student union and RADA. I am in the heart of London University and it feels like it, leafy Georgian Squares with faded facades and dim buildings now rather wrecked inside by cheap university carpets, fluorescent lights and nasty cream walls, saved by the presence of brilliant minds.

Waterstones is on the corner. After my blood tests, which don't take long, I go in there. Within twenty minutes I have spent £50. This could be an expensive autumn.

Friday, 20 September

I don't want to go to UCLH tomorrow for chemotherapy. I don't want a stem cell harvest. I don't want to remember I have cancer. I don't want to be that person. I cry. But before I cry, I go to the service at which our plaque to P.G. Wodehouse, long-awaited, is unveiled in Westminster Abbey, and laugh out loud at Alexander Armstrong's impression of Jeeves.

Saturday, 21 September

I cycle along my lovely London route dressed up for the chemotherapy with my pearls and lipstick, and arrive, shoulders braced, at an eerily quiet Cancer Centre. I go to the second floor where, during the week, chemotherapy is infused in patients in a large open space, airy and light but very exposed to the stares of passing people. It is deserted now, apart from one lady, possibly a cleaner, pushing a trolley, walking away from me. Then I see one man in a chemotherapy chair (grey, rather smarter than Guy's), hooked up to a drip, but he has his eyes closed and I don't want to disturb him. Then another person who could be a patient or a clinician walks past and I ask him for directions. He takes me along a corridor in the far corner of this vast atrium, and suddenly I am in a rather claustrophobic side-room with about six people having chemotherapy. They look quite ill, all of them.

'There's another cycloprime waiting,' says one of the nurses, seeing me. I'm the 'cycloprime': Cyclophosphamide priming for the stem cell harvest.

A lady in the corner quietly pukes.

I have never seen such a fat bag of chemotherapy as mine. Before May I'd never seen a bag of chemotherapy at all, but I'm familiar now and this is enormous. Oh Lord, more poison. I've been having Cyclophosphamide, as you will remember, Dear Readers, alongside Carfilzomib, but nothing like this amount. Just before the chemo, a 'push', as it's called, a quick infusion, of Mesa (I think that's its name) which does something to the Cyclophosphamide to stop it making my bladder bleed. Nice. I have to take some more Mesa, in tablet form, later, as well as more Ondansetron – glory be to God, not for 'dappled things' today, but for strong anti-emetics.

After it's all over – Seán brings me a huge bunch of sunflowers – the over-chatty taxi driver picks us up outside the Cancer Centre. He asks, 'What have you been doing this morning, then?' I say, 'Having chemotherapy.' I think he won't be surprised, given the location, but it upsets him. Seán, as ever, saves the day, and they chat amicably while I breathe the Saturday London air through my open window.

We stagger down to Hastings. I listen to *Our Mutual Friend* through my gorgeous rose-gold earphones and look at the scenery, which is still beautiful, but seems a little tired, ready for a change, showing autumnal hints. I feel light-headed, but not sick.

Sunday, 22 September

I am obliged once more to honour the sabbath. I don't feel sick. I don't feel sick! But I have slept badly for two nights and I am full of poison (honestly, that bag was enormous and it's all in me). I reflect how quickly I dropped the notion of a day with no oughts in it when it was no longer forced upon me by my physical state. I reverted, in my month away from chemotherapy, to my old self, and now I am grumpy at my personal change of season, from a brief summer's respite to autumn's gruelling . . . well I won't know exactly what gruelling until around 21 October when the randomisation happens, but there's plenty of gruelling in the meantime.

I start my week of SELF-INJECTED granulocyte-colony stimulating factor (Zarzio), to be administered daily until the stem cell harvest next Monday. Oh heavens! The nurse yesterday, who was in a bit of a hurry, showed me what to do, only she didn't really. She got me to pinch the skin on her arm, which is what you're meant to do to your stomach before injecting, then she said I was hurting her. I said I was nervous. Then I vaguely pointed the scary syringe at her pinched-up skin, but since it was still in its blister pack I didn't learn anything about how it worked. That was my practice.

I take the first needle out of the fridge at 5.30pm, as instructed, so that the Zarzio can warm up a bit before going into me. 'Otherwise it will sting,' said clinical nurse specialist Jackie, who is in charge of me for this next treatment. Seán and I sit either side of the kitchen table, the syringe between us, and distract ourselves with conversation. I look at the clock constantly. I am really nervous.

Finally 6.00pm strikes and we go next door into the main room — it seems appropriate not to do it in the kitchen — and then I don't know whether to sit or lie or stand. I sit. I forget I'm supposed to pinch my stomach and look despairingly down at it, over my drawn-up clothes; I can't really see it properly. I'm anxious and sleep deprived. I take the syringe out of its blister pack and take off its plastic top, revealing . . . the needle. Bugger. I thought it would be like a pen and I could just hold it against my stomach and not see the needle at all. I realise that I have always looked away when I've been injected, had bloods taken, been cannulated. I don't like needles. I put the needle against my skin but I still have it in my head that by pushing the blue plunger all the work will be done – the needle going in, the Zarzio being injected. I think Seán is telling me to do something but I am fixated on manipulating the plunger. 'Press it until it clicks, then let go, and the needle will retract,' the nurse had said. So I do. I have my eyes closed, and I feel liquid on my fingers. I'm bleeding. I can't look. Seán says, you've pulled it out. I say, I haven't done anything. When I'm sure I can't push the plunger any further I let go. I open my eyes. No blood. The liquid I can feel is the Zarzio that's meant to be inside me, that didn't go in because I didn't push the needle into my stomach. But some went in, because there's a kind of bubble in my skin. What have I done? Has it gone in far enough, and how much went in?? Do I need to do it again? I go into the kitchen and count the needles. I have nine left: two spares. I could try again. It's Sunday night. I ring the nurse, but understandably she's not answering. Then Seán looks at the information leaflet which says, if you don't get it all in don't give yourself another dose. The itchy bubble on my stomach slowly subsides. Something has gone in.

It isn't a good idea to give yourself, or anyone else for that matter, an injection with your eyes closed.

I am disproportionately furious. No one said, push the needle into your skin. This is all new to me. I need step-by-step instruction, and a rehearsal. I wouldn't ask a nurse to give a lecture on ethics in Westminster Abbey without instruction and a rehearsal, would I?

Well I know now. Monday night's injection will be a star performance. It's a shame today wasn't a rehearsal. I'll try not to worry that I've not kick-started my stem cell growth as much as I should have done.

I sleep badly again – three hours awake between midnight and 3.00am, just the time when, according to Chinese medicine, my spleen and my liver are restored. My spleen is compromised by the Cyclophosphamide and my liver is working overtime to process the poison, and neither of them is being restored because I can't sleep. I feel hopeless and cry.

I feel like a child.

When I was a child I asked God for things I wanted. Now I ask God for sleep. Just that. Sleep.

Twenty-fourth Letter

Dear Readers

Tonight I am a positive pro with the needle. Seán is on the phone at the time I am to administer myself, so, rather piqued at his inattention, I nevertheless take the syringe out of its blister pack, and, with a deep breath, remove the plastic cover on the needle, and look at the needle until it ceases to horrify. I squeeze up a bit of my tummy and clean it with an alcohol wipe. And I insert the needle into my squidge. The needle is so fine that I am able to imagine it entering between skin cells and fatty cells; though there is an undoubted pk! puncture moment as it passes through my skin. Then I deliberately place my thumb on the blue plunger and press gently to send in the growth factor slowly, keeping pressing until the promised click makes the needle recede into the syringe. I lift it clear and place it in the little sharps bin I've been given, wipe my tummy again, and cover it up. Job done, as the young people say. Seán is still chatting on the phone, blissfully unaware of the drama on the other side of the room. I feel immensely proud of myself.

I will, however, never make a junkie, nor a pierced, tattooed person. It seems very strange, to pierce one's body. Though I do have pierced ears; and in a fit of rebellion at forty, accompanied by my astonished sister who supportively had hers done too, a long-disused piercing in my belly button.

Tuesday, 24 September

I sit in bed, feeling rotten. I have a cold. All those efforts to avoid infection haven't worked. I reluctantly but dutifully take my temperature but luckily it's not high enough to warrant drastic hospital action. But I feel ill, and the rain and the wind are beating against the house, and I think I am not going to be able to ride. What a blow.

When I'm not feeling well, nothing really matters except . . . well, nothing really matters. It's the same in the middle of the night if I can't sleep. It's wretched, a kind of meaninglessness descends. You hope rather than believe that something of value is happening. And you just have to wait until you feel better.

Thursday, 26 September

I wasn't able to go to mass last Sunday because of the post-chemotherapy unwellness. Seán told me that Fr Eamonn said his blessing of Seán was a blessing for me too.

If you are not a Catholic, you can't receive the bread and wine at Communion in a Catholic church. So when I go up to the altar with everyone else to receive Communion, they get a consecrated wafer, the body of Christ, and I get a blessing because I'm an Anglican.

Now admittedly it's a bit excluding. But the blessings I've received in the place of the body of Christ have been wonderful. Fr Eamonn describes a cross on my forehead and blesses me in the name of the Father, the Son and the Holy Spirit, and I *feel* blessed. It is a holy moment, an eternal one, a piercing through time and space to a place of benediction.

In Ireland I make priests' lives complicated by going up with everyone at Communion and asking for a blessing. In Catholic countries this is unusual, and quite often the priest will try and poke a wafer into my resisting mouth. Trying to keep my mouth closed not to receive the wafer and at the same time explain that I'm Anglican and could I have a blessing please is complicated; when everyone else just passes through, seamlessly receiving, not holding up the proceedings. In Cork, after our mini-altercation, the elderly priest put the wafer back in the ciborium and clutched my arm. 'Yer all right,' he said, squeezing it. That was my blessing. It is the best blessing I've ever had, and I often remember it. *Yer all right.*

Friday, 27 September

A gap in the rain means we can ride. It is glorious, windy, sunny. The horses are calmed by a long trot to begin with, to use up some of their energy, and our first canter is uphill on a narrow lane, which instills some discipline, so the longer canter along the dell in the middle of the big field which can get a bit wild isn't too wild. I am on Nutkin who is comfortable and energetic today. When she walks fast, she reminds me of the bouncy walk of a toddler who naturally uses all its little body and its feet in the walk. That's how we should walk, Glenda tells us in Pilates. Not stiffen up. Nutkin bounces and cradles and rocks me in a jolly and nurturing way.

Windy autumn! Back in the warm, I listen to the rain swish against the house, watch the pearly light and the grey-green sea whipped into lively waves which break and re-form, white horses as far as the eye can see.

I feel no stem cells growing. Nor do I appear to be growing anything else, an extra digit or another head or anything. So I hope the chemotherapy and the injections are working. I look at my arms and wonder, from time to time, what's going on in there. I keep thinking of super-ovulation in IVF. But I'm not producing eggs for new life. This is entirely self-interested.

Saturday, 28 September

We have lovely massage and sacro-cranial treatment from Samvida, who says she can feel a lot of fluidity in my central nervous system, and it doesn't feel inflamed but natural. Is my bone marrow starting to produce? As I walk back along the front, watching the lively waves, my hair whipped by the wind, I feel a tremendous sense of well-being. I walk bouncily, like Nutkin and toddlers. But then later I feel pain. Over our fish-and-chip supper it worsens, to sharp electric spasms that make me catch my breath. Is this the bone pain promised by the stem cell over-production? I think of the contractions preceding childbirth (for 'contractions' read 'nearly unbearable pain') and like those, this sharp pain recedes and returns. It is crippling while it lasts, hard to think of anything else. How awful to have it for any length of time. Awful. I take paracetamol and have a deep, hot bath with lots of Epsom salts dissolved in the water, and I go to bed. The pain doesn't return until the middle of the night; I take more paracetamol and it recedes again.

Sunday, 29 September

The rather Platonic relationship with my body that I inherited from my youthful indoctrination was summed up in a kind of mantra we were taught: 'I am not this body, it is an instrument for my use'. But the pain makes me understand that I am my body.

The harvest is tomorrow. Think of me, Dear Readers, for a moment, if you remember, in the morning. I will be for five hours hooked up to a machine. Let's hope I produce 276 million cells in one session; otherwise I have to give myself another injection and go back for more the next day . . .

Twenty-fifth Letter

Dear Readers

Monday, 30 September

I have another bad night but stagger out of bed at 6.00am to prepare myself for the stem cell harvest. I have to think about what to wear: my dress has to be easily adjustable in case I need to use a bed pan during the procedure, since I can't be unhooked from the harvesting machine during the five hours it is going to take. I end up choosing a dress I last wore to meet the Queen, believe it or not: navy blue, Phase Eight, with an elasticated waist, which is cool and surprisingly flattering. That bucks me up. I love the idea of dressing up to go to hospital. Both the NHS and the Queen merit honour.

I eat breakfast much earlier than I care to; and drink my required litre of water as quickly as I can: I really do not want to need the lavatory all morning. Beginning to run out of time, I hastily prepare a little pile of overnight things for Seán to collect as there is just a chance I am kept in overnight. I spend far too long dithering over the task (dressing gown? nightshirt?? mascara???) and which books to bring. I have my rose-gold earphones and *Silas Marner* to listen to. Finally, I am ready and head off with a loaded bag to the hospital.

I choose to cycle, riding high on the imaginative and moving messages of support from you, Dear Readers. (I can smell the candle you have lit, dear S.) It's not raining, and I will be lying still for a long time, so I want the exercise and I try to enjoy the journey. I check the north side panorama of the Thames as I cross Waterloo Bridge and, no, I cannot see the dome and statue of Justice atop the Old Bailey. I can see St Martin-in-the-Fields' spire, though, with its blue clock, now set to atomic time since it was refurbished, and its exquisite gold weathervane right at the pinnacle, where a huge Pride flag flew during the celebrations.

As I cycle, prompted by your observation that my personal harvest is happening at harvest tide, C, I sing 'We Plough the Fields and Scatter'.

I arrive and find what I think is the harvest room. I ask if this is where one comes if one wants a stem cell harvest and am not found very funny. There are seven beds in the room, with a squat R2D2-like machine beside each. I am allocated one of the beds and discover that my machine is called Rosie. The one beside the adjacent bed is Apollo. They all have what look like big keys sticking out of their fronts, as though you could wind them up. I climb on my bed; then I notice a lady opposite with her man companion whom I'd seen and smiled at last week when I had my Cyclophosphamide. Always on the lookout for more Cardamon trial participants, I go over and introduce myself. E is not in Cardamon but she does have myeloma. Her machine is called Aphrodite and I'm a bit jealous. Between being weighed, having our height, blood pressure, temperature and pulse rate measured, and having blood tests to see if we are likely to produce stem cells for harvesting today, E, L her husband and I fall into a quiet but passionate argument about. Yes. E voted remain, L voted leave. L thinks that the EU is the sign of the anti-Christ (I have a feeling a significant number of people think this). They are both very rude about MPs and that, Dear Readers, is what I cannot stop myself from heatedly denying. I can avoid arguments about Brexit but I cannot stand by and hear perfectly intelligent people dismiss our MPs as, severally, useless, corrupt, children, in it for themselves, lining their pockets, sitting back and doing nothing, etc., etc. We are each speaking quietly, but quickly, and with a staccato rhythm, and mostly all at the same time, rather enjoying it. But we bring ourselves down from the ceiling in time — E and I are meant to be staying calm, ready for our ordeal, after all — and E tells me how she copes with her cancer with a clearly deep faith in God that shines out of her eyes when she speaks of it, far more confidently than I ever could. She is beautiful and young and vibrant, and like me, she has dressed well for hospital in a bright spangly top. L is mellow with dreadlocks and a hat. We part on excellent terms.

Our blood test results come back and I am recalled to my bed. I don't know what these numbers mean but am nevertheless competitive. E has ninety-four and I have 194, good numbers both, indicating a bumper harvest. My neighbour in the bed with Apollo has, appropriately, 300. We all pop to the loo several times to try and empty our bladders but mine seizes up (though thank you, M, for running water images).

I then suffer a long, painful episode of vein-hunting. The biggest vein, on my left arm, is reserved for the taking out of blood to go into Rosie, but a vein has to be found in my right arm to put the blood back. 'Used and abused', the nurse says of my veins. She tries three times, Dear Readers, and when I write 'try' I mean: taps my arm, finds a possible vein, cleans the area, 'deep breath', pokes in the cannula, ouch, pushes it in further, ouch, further, OUCH, as it hits a valve, and then frustratedly out again. I'm told that it's not just used and abused veins that make cannulation difficult, but also that my blood is thick with white blood cells now.

Here is a metaphor to play with: you may be full to the brim with something you want to give (love, say) but your vessels are too small to let it out. Or the world may be full of something you want to receive (love, say) but your vessels are too small to let it in. And sometimes the size or bulk or substantiveness of the thing is what overwhelms the vessels. Should we work on enlarging our vessels (can we)? Should we accept their size and be patient, giving and receiving at the pace they set? Blood: love: life: exchange and movement: they have to flow.

Eventually, a more senior nurse is called in to help. Consuelo manages to find a vein at the fourth attempt. But the only workable vein is in the crook of my elbow. You cannot move the arm from which the blood is being taken during the harvesting, but the arm which is receiving the blood back is usually mobile. Not when the cannula is in my elbow. So I am obliged to lie with both arms straight out either side of me, for the whole proceedings. My book-dithering is rendered pointless as I will not be able to scratch my nose, let alone hold a book and turn its pages.

When all choice is taken from you, you can surrender, I discover, with considerable relief, to the one course of action left. Clara, a new nurse on the block and very tender and smily, kindly arranges my rose-gold headphones over my ears and I tap my phone at the end of my right arm to call up *Silas Marner*, and I close my eyes and relax into lying absolutely still, listening to George Eliot's marvellous cadences, quiet descriptions, gentle characterisation and deep, simple wisdom. And nod off. When I awake, Seán is here. I have some hot water on my table, and he gives me some sips, removes my headphones and we chat for a while.

Then the inevitable (for me: everyone else seems to have stronger bladders) need for the lavatory. Consuelo brings me a commode. Another new experience to face up to and . . . just accept. The nurse pulls the curtains round and helps me off the bed ensuring I don't bend my arms. She adjusts my dress. I had removed my knickers earlier to keep things simple, thank heavens, and once I am settled on the thing I am left alone, and I watch Rosie do her rumbling work. It's fine. It's really fine, quite nice actually. It's noisy outside the curtain so I have no bladder shyness. Seán has sight of my bottom as I am helped off the commode and back on to the bed. He has of course seen it many times, but this is so immensely unsexy. He is gorgeous about it. 'You still have one,' he reassures me.

And so the morning wears on, Rosie chuntering beside me, *Silas Marner* in my ears. Seán feeds me with some tuna sandwiches and a bit more water and, most delicious of all, juicy orange segments. He scratches my nose when it itches. I try to do 'still Pilates'. I work with my imagination through the muscles of my body, starting with my feet, and it feels like proper relieving exercise.

Daniel, who is I think in charge of the unit, comes over with Clara to explain how Rosie works and I listen to the masterclass.

Well. This £250k-machine receives and processes all of my blood two-and-a-half times. Before the blood enters the machine, it is joined by anti-coagulant. In it goes, where it is spun, and then through one very fine tube emerges salmon-pink blood which is deposited in a drip bag. These are the stem cells. The see-through tube blood passes over what looks like paint colour samples to ensure the fluid is the right shade of pink, otherwise something is wrong.

Stem cells are medium weight while red blood cells are heavy and plasma is light, so Rosie separates the stem cells by their relative weight. Another big tube of pale blood is returned to me through my other obediently straight arm. I watch, fascinated and rather spooked as my blood leaves me and comes back to me. Two-and-a-half times. It's like draining the plumbing system of your house.

I have been relieved to be told that only two million stem cells per kilogram of body weight are needed, not four million as I had understood. So that's only 138 million stem cells. I am further relieved to hear that my weight has been adjusted downwards to sixty kilograms because that's about right for my height (oh dear), so the amount needed goes down again to 120 million stem cells.

At one point, Seán and I talk about the stability and wealth needed to make this privileged medicine possible. I feel the grotesque unfairness that I should have a £250k-machine all to myself for half a day, prolonging my life in relative comfort; if I was another human being on another part of the SAME PLANET I would not have any of this. I read your accounts of the situation in Zimbabwe, N, and shiver. I receive what I am offered, of course, but it is not just, and I cannot rejoice wholeheartedly in my own healthcare.

You know that feeling towards the end of a long-haul flight (when you're in steerage) when you've still an hour-and-a-half to go but because it has been so long that hour-and-a-half feels like the end of the journey, and you look again and again at the map of the world and the little image of the aeroplane moving across it to your destination, willing it to speed up and just land and let you stretch your limbs and breathe real air again? That's what my ordeal becomes. (Not, obviously, if you're travelling business class, when you simply order more champagne and rather hope the journey won't end too soon. And listen to me, describing another privileged experience to explain this one.) I watch my little bag of stem cells grow in volume. Collected in the drip bag they are no longer salmon pink but rich, thick red, like tomato ketchup. What volume does 120 million stem cells look like?

Eventually, I am given a four-minute warning, after which the big cannula in my left arm, by now aching quite badly, is taken out. A tourniquet applied over the bandage means I still can't bend my arm.

My other arm is receiving the last of my blood but then Consuelo ties the tube off which still has some of my blood in it; I watch, a tad worried. Don't I need that blood? Consuelo says I won't miss it. She leaves the cannula in my arm, telling me it might be needed for more blood (someone else's?) or drugs if I don't recover properly.

I am allowed to visit the lavatory but have to return to have my vitals measured again. My blood pressure is eighty over something. But I hadn't felt faint when I walked to the loo so we try the other machine. 104. Mmm. That's high enough to let me go home, but the difference between the two machines isn't reassuring. But I feel fine, and anyway we have to wait until the results of the harvest are known, since if there aren't enough I have to come back tomorrow, heaven help me. We go to have tea in the main foyer of the Cancer Centre on the ground floor. I realise I am sporting a bloody cannula in my right arm, the sort of spectacle that has become so normal to me now but would have freaked me out if I'd seen it the first time I entered the Cancer Centre at Guy's, and when I think of this (rather late on) I cover it with my scarf.

After forty-five minutes we return to the unit. Already the beds are occupied with a new set of patients. E and L have gone. My results come through. There's a sort of gasp and cheer from the nurse looking at her computer. '14.2,' she says. 'You've produced 7.2 times more stem cells than you need.' That is, I've produced, my brilliant responsive body has produced, 852 million stem cells. I ask the lady in the bed by me if she would like some. 'Surely someone can use the spares?' I plead with the staff. Seems not.

With that strange proud feeling that comes from having done not very much myself but having pleased the clinical staff, Seán and I totter out of the Centre and fall into a taxi.

Later, on my own, I sob my heart out. Needless to say, I am depleted in all sorts of ways, physically and psychologically. My blood is recovering from its two-and-a-half trips into Rosie, and my blood pressure is probably still low, but I don't want a pill to sort me out. I want to feel this. I'm sad and overwrought. I went through a lot today. I feel as though I have been assaulted. I was pinned to the bed, helpless; Seán giving me sips of water; Consuelo helping me on to the commode. It was fine, of course it was fine, and everyone was lovely, but I am left feeling as though something has been taken from me.

My freedom.

Just for five hours, in a good cause, and I have it back now and I will recover. But for that time I was a prisoner and I think that is why I am weeping, and that makes me think about the value I place upon freedom and willpower and selfhood. Take away my autonomy and I feel my humanity denuded. Of course our fallibility brings out good things in others, given the right context, like hospitals. And I do not believe we are really autonomous because we are subject to so many forces outside our own control. But most of the time, if you are healthy, you feel autonomous enough to experience freedom. You can intend to act and then act.

The funny thing is that while I was undergoing the harvest, pinned to the bed, keeping quite still, I was content. I really didn't mind being fed and watered and so on. It is only afterwards that I weep. Is it that, in order to cope, the enclosed human spirit and body shrinks into a smaller space than the one imprisoning it, in order not to feel constrained? I assented to my circumstances and found my peace within them. Being still is quite relaxing, as is letting others care for your physical needs. If I pursue the analogy of shrinking oneself to fit within the constraints of one's circumstances, how do I know that I am not doing that right now, it's just that the constraints are much looser? In the UK the constitution protects freedoms; we are constrained by the law but its circumference is, for the most part, so far away that we operate quite happily within it. In a country where such freedoms are not protected, the constraints are much closer. Perhaps then the temptation to live a really small life is all the greater, because if you tried to do bigger, more public service type things, you'd feel the constraints and have to do something about them.

Friday, 4 October

I ride Nutkin. I do love her. I sense her intelligence though I don't know how to read it. At a certain point in the ride I realise just how connected I am to her physically: I can't quite tell where my legs stop and her strong back starts. It's a wonderful feeling; as though we are one body, like a centaur (well not quite, because I'm on top, not in front, but perhaps that's where the centaur idea comes from). I remember watching a cowboy ride into the distance when I stayed on a 'dude ranch' in Arizona. He and the horse were one. Why is it so exquisitely beautiful to see that, and so particularly wonderful to feel it now on Nutkin?

The ground is wet and the horses struggle through mud around the edge of one of the big fields. The machinery, ploughing the field, has trimmed the trees and hedges on its way past. I look sadly at the clumsily torn and snapped-off branches. A human hand would have done that so much more sympathetically, attending to the health of the plant, not just the space created by trimming it.

Saturday, 5 October

I meet A, one of Hastings' many colourful characters, outside Mel's in the High Street, and she tells me how well I look, better than I ever have done. I wonder if my face isn't reflecting a (kind of) peace of mind, borne of having to face invasive treatments and tests and overcome my fear, again and again, and above all of having to face death, every morning once more remembering that I have cancer and that I am going to die. But I don't want to lie passively pinned to my destiny like I was pinned to Rosie. I don't want to surrender the ambition which I still harbour, to be counted among the great women of Balliol, my old college, whose celebration of its fortieth anniversary of admitting women I have had to miss. Yes, dear A, if I am alive, I will go with you to the fiftieth anniversary.

Twenty-sixth Letter

Dear Readers

Sunday, 6 October

I watch my hair worriedly. It is two weeks since my Cyclophosphamide infusion, and F's hair fell out at this point. I am definitely shedding more. I was promised thinning, not losing it altogether, and F said her clinician swore she had never seen it happen before so it should be safe. It should be. I meditate on tightly closed apertures in my scalp, holding on to my hair. Sometimes porosity is not what is wanted. Sometimes I have to hang on to what is in me and with me, for protection, self-worth, in order to be someone who can learn and be open to others. Not wholly dependent upon the love and acclaim that others give me, but strong in myself too. Today my hair seems to be part of that.

I pluck my eyebrows, which are growing where the tattoos are not. Are the hairs easier to pluck? I'm not sure.

Monday, 7 October

Hanks of hair coming out in my hands in the bath and at the sink. 'More is on my head than is coming off,' I keep muttering, my heart hammering as the ball of hair grows and grows. I didn't wash my hair yesterday. Would washing it make things worse? Or just reveal the inevitable? This morning I have to wash it and my bath swims with hair. I who cannot bear a single hair dallying in the bathroom, or on my clothes, or anywhere apart from people's heads, I who am avid about clearing up my own hair mess in a bathroom, I am *wading* through hair. I am just as avid cleaning up now, but the task is Herculean. My Augean stable keeps filling up as more hairs fall from my head, catch in my comb, settle in the sink. Hercules had a day; I have a train to catch. I don't know if I am making things worse by washing it but once I have started I can't stop: I have to comb it out; I have to dress it. I am as gentle as my shaking hands can be. Eventually it is done, and it looks normal. You wouldn't notice. But I have handfuls of hair to show Seán. He suggests an artist might make something of it, and we remember Mona Hatum, whose enormous installations featured quantities of hair twisted and woven and turned into rope and curtain. I like the metaphor but hate the reality — I really dislike her work. I think of concentration camps and the use that inmates' hair was put to after their heads had been shaven. The only place for my great switch of hair is in the compost, making new life. I hope it does.

I think, this is a good rehearsal. It is such a shock; and if I have the stem cell transplant and it all falls out, I have had a taste of what that is like. It cannot be hidden, you see. Everything else I have gone through is on the inside: I can hide away during the sickness; put make up and a smile on my face. I've enjoyed being told how well I look; defiant in the face of the challenge of cancer. But everyone will see the hair loss. And however quickly my friends will get used to how I look, the initial view is a shock and for the general public, baldness on women is just weird.

Tuesday, 8 October

Already I am adjusting to the (continuing) loss of my hair. I still have so much on my head. I will ride this. I tell myself I'm a 'strong lass' as you say, S.

I read Jocelyn Playfair's *House in the Country*,[4] which is set during the Second World War . The characters are idealistic about the future and how to avoid war; they are unhappy at the willingness of people to return as quickly as they can to their quotidian lives. Living a small life means you avoid feeling the constraints visited upon you, as I discovered during the stem cell harvest. But it's also true that that same pedestrian concentration on small things was one of the ways in which the country survived during conflict. Getting up and dressed and having a cup of tea. Are families in Syria and other war-torn places finding something strong in their attempts to live their everyday lives in the midst of chaos and fear?

Today I have another bone marrow biopsy, one of the tests that has to be done before randomisation. It is as vile as ever; really the worst thing. No, not the worst thing. Losing my hair is the worst thing. Or is it the nausea? So many worst things! The biopsy is of both the aspirate and the trefoil: the honey and the honeycomb. The latter involves cutting out actual bone structure and is horrible. I take paracetamol and co-codamol, which are not meant to be taken together, and I have gas and air, which I suck on with abandon. No hanging on to control this time. And I do enter a strange place of not caring. The doctor who is doing the procedure this time is very experienced and lovely in a surgeon kind of a way, which is to say, not very human, but highly competent and trustworthy. He has a new doctor with him, watching the procedure, and he explains what he is doing. I am interested to begin with but then I cease to care, I just want it to end. I shout at the pain. Afterwards I see the implements. They are enormous metal chisel-like things with handles to screw round and bore into the bone and take out the samples. I feel retrospectively faint.

The dreadful randomisation decision is about to be made. All the needful tests are complete. It's like waiting for an exam result that will affect your whole life.

I try to maintain equilibrium by reminding myself that we — the clinicians and I — are all in equipoise over the two arms of the trial. The transplant, which I dread, is nevertheless the gold standard; the consolidation Carfilzomib, which I want, is experimental and may not work as well; we do not know which is better. Both give me equal chances of survival, as far as anyone knows, but (my equilibrium failing) I think: the treatment experience will be dramatically different. The transplant is like death and rebirth, the Carfilzomib is a less exciting endurance test. The Carfilzomib will allow me to retain some semblance of my old self; I will look the same. It is a repeat of the induction chemotherapy regime and I believe I can cope with it; at least I know from experience what it entails. The transplant may be transformative, taking me to a new place in myself entirely. Then I think: if I have consolidation Carfilzomib my Dear Reader letters will become boring. That, weirdly, helps me mind less if I am randomised to the transplant. Better material!

I can do nothing to influence the decision. It is a lottery, but a fair one; either way I 'win'. But whichever treatment I am allocated, I'll look at the other one and wonder if I'd be better off with it.

All the rationalising doesn't help the horrible, horrible feeling of dread as I wait.

My hair is STILL coming out in great hanks, wafting about the bathroom, creating great drifts on the floor. I can't believe I still look normal.

Wednesday, 9 October

I wash my hair and even more of it comes out. It fills the bathroom dustbin. I cry. Every time I put my hand to my head a lock of hair comes away.

I feel dreadfully self-conscious and out of sorts. I don't want to go out, but it's choir night, and I make myself. I am initially prickly with my friends, but their great kindness melts my defensive shell and I relax into a new vulnerable self, allowing the gentle choir world in, letting them look after me instead of holding up a strong but clearly brittle self that can no longer rely upon part of what I think I am: my appearance. And starting with the choir, I can surrender to the glances rather than flinching away from them. I can practise interosculating.

Thursday, 10 October

I keep having to rein in my imagination when it sees me randomised to Carfilzomib, delighted at the lesser of two evils, able to be (nearly) myself again – but who is the self I wish to return to? Haven't I been transformed already? Wouldn't I be pretending, trying to return to a pre-cancer Claire by whom no one is deceived?

Hair still looses itself from the anchor of my head and falls from me. I don't like to comb it, since just touching precipitates greater shedding. Does God really count every hair? I'm impressed.

Many people in middle age suffer hair thinning. I was irritated at Amber Rudd's messy hair, but maybe she avoided combing it because it, too, was falling out.

And nature is fecund, I ponder as I look at my head which still looks all right. What was all that spare hair for?

I am depressed by a brief conversation with my French neighbour, who positions herself as 'us' Europeans and me as 'you' British not making our Brexit minds up. 'Stay or go,' she says. I don't want to be on the side she has placed me. But I am not separate from my fellow citizens.

10.30am

I receive an email from Sarah, clinical trial practitioner, to say that she has sent my form to the place where the randomisation happens. She says it usually takes three hours. So I should know in three hours' time which arm of the trial I am in.

Jesus, dear Lord Jesus, grant me equilibrium. I feel sick. I can't help it. Wouldn't you: knowing your fate for the next six months is about to be sealed? The trauma of hair thinning has made it worse: my poor denuded scalp still resembles 'me' but it won't, it *won't* if I have the transplant.

I desperately think about making the Cotton Rooms (the 'hotel' where we stay if we have the transplant) a good experience. Shall I start a jigsaw in the lounge so all the guests can have a go? Or would that be too infection-liable?

I need the loo.

I'm breathing deeply.

My heart is rattling in my ribcage.

I have put a smile on my face. Yesterday on Radio 4 Bill Bryson read from his book on the human body that we can make our lips smile but we cannot manufacture smiling eyes.

I look in the mirror, smiling with all my might. My eyes are all crinkled up but they don't look as though they're smiling. They look scared. And . . . a little bit excited, eager even.

I turn consciously towards this next step. I embrace it now, whatever it is. I am willing to feel whatever I am going to feel, to the tips of my everything, body, mind, heart and spirit.

I am comforted by writing out this passage from Julian's eleventh revelation, Mary's experience kindling a deep kind of hope:

> My lord showed me nothing in special but our lady saint Mary, and her he showed three times. The first was as she conceived, the second was in her sorrows under the cross, and the third was as she is now, in liking, worship and joy . . . Wilt thou see in her how thou art loved?

Sarah's email arrives with the decision.

I am to have the transplant.

So the worst has happened and I'm still upright. I am not now letting myself think, for one moment (well just one, briefly), about what might have been, about the fact that my life might have resembled something relatively close to normal if the result had gone the other way.

I determine this: even as my bone marrow is destroyed by the killer chemotherapy Melphalan and my stem cells returned to me for my rebirth, I will let myself be transformed in my spiritual marrow. I determine that this will be an experience to relish and be changed by, for the better; not something to shrink from and wish away.

But, oh fuck fuck fuck fuck fuck fuck fuck fuck.

Hearing this feels worse than hearing the original diagnosis of cancer, believe it or not.

Friday, 11 October

How do you make a line shorter without doing anything to the line?

You draw a longer line next to it.

Now I'm not at all troubled by my hair falling out. There's no need to hang on to it. It falls like autumn leaves from a tree preparing for winter. It will all go, and in the spring it will return. It is not precious to me anymore, not this failing thatch.

My riding hat swivels on my head, now so much hair has gone. I ride L'Arcelle, and I think she can feel my discombobulation: she is as jumpy as am I. But it is a magnificent ride in the driving rain and buffeting wind; some stirring canters, and long heart-expanding views of hilly Sussex all the way to the shining sea. Once I have returned L'Arcelle to her stable and given her water, once I am out in the rain again and on my own, tears fall.

★   ★   ★

I reread the beginning of Julian. She conceived a wish, when she was young, that when she was thirty she should have an illness that would bring her so close to death that she would suffer all the pains associated with dying, and that she and all about her would believe that she was going to die. She would receive the last rites. She wished this in order to be purged by the mercy of God and 'after live more to the worship of God, because of that sickness'.

This sickness did indeed come upon her when she was 'thirty and a half'. As she lay in bed, so close to death, 'nothing was in earth that I liked to live for, nor for no pain that I was afeard of, for I trusted in God of his mercy'.

Help me, Julian, to embrace what is to come.

A concert of Mozart and Beethoven by Hastings Philharmonia (beautiful, beautiful young, talented musicians) is inexpressibly comforting, not least because I wear a soft brown velvet beret with a silk flower which I had bought from Mel at The Wardrobe some time back; it looks good!

Saturday, 12 October

Another day, another hat: I have bought a baker boy's hat with leopard skin spots and it is jaunty. I tuck all my surviving hair into it, so that it looks as it will do when I have no hair, and wear it to a private view. My skin glows from one of Elinor's yoga-for-the-face treatments; my feet smile from her pedicure and my toenails, though hidden, sport a subtle burnt orange colour. I am complimented on my appearance, although one acquaintance appears to be offended by my blooming looks, since that's not what cancer is supposed to bring. I have several loving and heartfelt conversations; and a reconciliation that is long overdue with a friend whom I think understands me only too well, which may be why we fell out in the first place. I enjoy learning how differently I see from P, who is an artist, who looks at one photograph and shows me the deep substantial, sooty quality of the surround; while I, a writer, am busy creating a story out of the shadowy figure behind the window in the middle of the picture.

A wig fitting has been arranged for me on Monday.

IV

Third Part of the Treatment

Twenty-seventh Letter

Dear Readers

I have a long conversation with D, a fellow myeloma patient, with whom Grace put me in touch, as she has had a stem cell transplant. She does not spare me any detail, for which I am grateful, but it is not easy to hear how bereft she felt of everything that made her feel normal; of her extreme helpless fatigue; of her weakness and vulnerability and negativity. And of the broken glass that coated her throat for days. Her hair was the least of her worries. And she says, 'Claire, it is worth it. You get through it.'

In shock after hearing this litany of challenges, I have a massage and cranio-sacral treatment from Samvida that soothes away the tight unhappy wrinkles in my soul.

I never take any notice of horoscopes (I always do), and today Shelley von Strunckel tells me:

> You've a knack for dealing with seriously tricky matters. However, those you are currently facing are forcing you to bow to an unknown destiny, which terrifies you. If you can't plunge in, think of the times in the past when you were equally anxious and things didn't just go well, those changes constituted long overdue breakthroughs. It's the same now.[1]

Monday, 14 October

I am thinking of the Extinction Rebellion protesters as I look out over a rain-soaked Old Town, the sea fast disappearing into the cloud, and hear the rain soft and thick, pattering on the canopy. I hope my fellow Londoners can roll with the protest, work around it, join it, acknowledge what it is presenting to them, and let it grant them a brief pause in their busy lives. Rather than see it as just another ruddy obstacle to stop them carrying on with their busy lives.

We speak, N, of the way in which being vulnerable evokes compassion in others, and gives others permission to be vulnerable themselves. But I don't want to be the vulnerable one. I don't want to be the one evoking pity; or if I am, then only in certain safe environments, on my own terms, and with a plan to make my way out of my weakness. I don't want to be weak.

But I am not weak, not at the moment anyway. I am thinking about how I will face the transplant. I am interpreting it as my own Julian experience. I am not just going to get through it as best I can, flinching from pain and misery. I shall enter it deeply, as Julian willingly faced her death and had her visions. I don't expect I'll have visions but the meaning of what I experience will be, for me, spiritual. Even if the only thing I can do when it is all at its worst is name the pain God, I shall do that. God not separate or different from whatever happens in this time; God in and through it. 'Nothing was in earth that I liked to live for, nor for no pain that I was afeard of, for I trusted in God of his mercy.' Call me mad, but I am energised by these thoughts. Now I am walking towards the experience with firm, not shrinking, steps. I am entering my own anchorhold, as Julian entered hers. I am going to die to the world.

When you are falling; dive.

I wash my hair, which has not stopped coming out in handfuls. You just have to last me one more week, I tell the follicles firmly, just one week of events at Westminster Abbey I am intending to go to; then I can step back from that smart world, wear jaunty caps or maybe the wig if it is ready, in Hastings, preparing for the huge tunnel of hard things to come that is the transplant.

But when I dry my hair, it is so fine and thin that it tangles into a matted lump that is impossible to comb out. I am immediately transported back to my childhood when my fine hair did just this whenever it was washed, my mother hurried and distracted by a thousand other tasks as the time to leave for school approached and I looked a fright. I apply a bottleful of conditioner, Seán helps, wielding the shower nozzle, but it is impossible to unknit the knot. Unlike the schoolgirl, and unlike me before I had the news of the transplant, I am mercifully detached from this head of hair; only concerned that no one will be able to fit a wig over the accidental dreadlock top knot I now sport. I squeeze it dry as well as I can and put on my baker boy cap which is baggy enough to cover the lump.

I look at myself in the mirror, enquiringly. This tangle has precipitated the moment, but I am ready.

Ready to shave it all off.

I am to be shriven *before* I enter my anchorhold.

We arrive in London in time to go to the barbers I have in mind, a friendly looking place on Newcomen Street we walk past every time I go to the Cancer Centre. It is a gentlemen's barbers, the shop front says, so, disappointed, we move on to a new barber which has opened up almost next door. That is also a gentlemen's barbers and it is peopled by sharp-faced beautiful young men doing clever sculpting things to other sharp-faced beautiful young men: not a place I can approach with my cancer-induced request. We return to the friendly looking barber. Encouraged by Seán, who is rightly convinced that for this task I need a barber's shaver, not scissors, I speak to the man at the desk who has a kind face. 'I am not a gentleman,' I say, 'but I have to shave my hair off because it's falling out anyway from chemotherapy. I have cancer.' His face softens even more and he says of course, and ushers me to a chair. I remove my cap and reveal the ruination of my head of hair. Seán sits in quiet attendance.

Then this angel of a man gently, oh so gently, shaves my head, carefully approaching the tangled knot, working his way over the contours of my scalp, leaving an inch of hair. which is mercifully still evenly distributed, a silver grey, revealing my head, revealing me.

I look at myself in the mirror and I see that I am fine. I am revealed, and what is revealed is just fine. I don't mean the appearance of me exactly, more that with nothing covering me, nothing to hide behind or pretend with, entirely on show, I am nothing to be ashamed of. I feel as vulnerable as I have ever felt, but I am also strangely relieved and liberated.

I am fine; until a customer who has witnessed the proceedings while having his own (prolific) hair cut walks past me on his way out and says, 'You look even better than when you came in. More bad-ass.' And then I dissolve into tears, and the beautiful angel – Al – quietly continues to give an artistic finish to my shaven head. We begin to speak to each other; I tell him a bit about my cancer, he tells me a bit about himself. He is Kurdish. His heart is breaking over what is happening to his people in northern Syria. I tell him about the wondrous Azad Cudi with whom I appeared on *Start the Week*, all those months ago just after my diagnosis. Al says someone, a Kurd who had been a sniper like Azad, was assassinated in London just a couple of weeks ago, by a gang of men Al thinks was ISIS. Was it Azad? We don't know. He says Kurds are not safe: 'We are Muslims helping the West,' he says. 'That makes us a target for those who think we are betrayers.' We are in compassionate communion as Al carefully neatens my crop. What is happening to me is so utterly unimportant in the context of the continued destruction of his people. But the tender attention Al gives my hair is our place of communion. What I had dreaded with the deepest dread I had had in all this time since my cancer was diagnosed is become a transcend-ent experience in which I am attended by an angel of the first order. It is one of the best experiences of my life so far. I am profoundly blessed.

Al will not take payment.

I am just in time for my next appointment for the wig fitting. I walk proudly down Newcomen Street to the Cancer Centre with no hat, showing my shriven, blessed, sanctified head to the world. And of course no one turns a hair (ha).

The ladies in the wig shop are a delight. Leyla takes me into the little cubicle and seats me in front of a mirror with lights all around it, like an actor's dressing room. But before I sit down, I swear I see my hair, an exact copy of the hair I have just lost, on a wig stand on the shelf. Leyla finds a wig cap, which is a stocking like the ones one imagines a bank robber wears, only shorter, fitting over my hair area. Then she puts the wig on my head. It's a bit shiny, and the fringe is too long, but otherwise it could be the head of hair Judith my hairdresser produces for me when I see her. I am astonished by how much I look like myself. Leyla expertly shortens and softens the fringe, and we are done. That quickly.

Tuesday, 15 October

My wig has its first outing: processing in my red cassock and black gown for the service at Westminster Abbey to mark the 750th anniversary of the building of the Henry III church. If you hadn't been so encouraging, L, I might not have come. But I do. I even cycle to the Abbey in my wig. In at the deep end, as public a first outing as I could have imagined. And only those who know my story guess it is a wig. I feel confident and warm. Thank heavens winter is coming. The wig feels like a snugly fitting cap. ('How come Claire's hair looks so healthy, with all the treatment she's having?' a colleague asks later.)

I undertake to sign the Institute's million (as it seems) Christmas cards as I won't be certain of having the energy to do so in late November. For this task I replace my wig with my baker boy cap for comfort; that in itself requires a deliberate and conscious choice to show my colleagues, not my bared head (yet), but a head clearly shaven under the cap. I am fessing to the wig. I'm glad to have options, glad I have colleagues whose loving support means that I have options.

(No one is really bothered.)

Easing my shoulder, arm and fingers out of their cramps from signing, I make my way to the National Gallery. I want the sustenance of great art before my incarceration. I spend a long time, nearly half an hour, in front of Rembrandt's *Portrait of an Old Woman*. His dark, velvety depth of humanity, unflinching characterisation of age and personality, her fearless wise gaze directly at me, the simplicity of it, the human reality of it, feed my soul. Then I stand for just as long in front of Leonardo's *Virgin on the Rocks*, and my soul is fed again, this time by the crystal clarity of his portrayal; its purity, its this-world-other-world gossamer thinness; I look at the Madonna's hand hovering over her child like the dove-Holy Spirit hovering as it does at his baptism; she blesses him, and he in turn blesses John the Baptist, but it could, I reflect, be the whole world.

Wednesday, 16 October

I stay late at the pub with my fellow choir members. I don't want to lose a minute of their company: next week is half term and I may not see them again until after Christmas.

You tell me, E, of your vision when you prayed for me, of the disciple whom Christ loved resting against him, his head reclining on Christ's shoulder (John 13:23). I am comforted.

Thursday, 17 October

I go with Seán to the Royal Academy for an inspiring afternoon. In the Antony Gormley exhibition I see a myriad depictions of the human form, the ways in which we stand, sit, lean against a wall, curl up on the floor, kneel, lie cruciform, hang from the ceiling and the walls, are spiky, porous, set in concrete, scarred, playful; we are encouraged to see ourselves as part of the exhibition as we move through. Never have I been so aware of my fellow humans in a gallery, where usually I am rather hoping they will all go away, ignoring them as I focus on the art, having my personal communion with it. Here the moving figures of the visitors interosculate with the exhibits and show new facets. I am struck, in the room of figures hanging from the walls and ceiling and standing on the floor, how they have been placed so as to have no connection at all with each other, as if each is occupying his own world and simply cannot see the other; and yet the flesh-and-blood visitors clump together, discussing the art, showing each other what they see. We are naturally gregarious; by contrast the scarred and rusting figures seem desolate to me.

There is a huge cuboid metal structure, different sized hollow squares stacked crazily atop each other. If you could look from above, we learn, you would see a human curled in the foetal position. We are invited to walk through. Seán enters and I meet him at the other side for a report; he encourages me but I hesitate, expecting claustrophobia. Strangely, I feel no little stabs of panic at the thought of enclosed spaces with people behind me blocking my escape (perhaps I have been hardened by all my claustrophobic hospital procedures), and so I venture forth, pulling back momentarily at the prospect of a very narrow, low passage, but launching again at it with the gallery assistant's voice echoing behind me: 'Feel the fear'. The squeezed space is mercifully short, and we emerge into a great chamber, just like the pyramids where you pass through what feels like a birth canal into an enormous chapel carved out of the rock (Seán tells me; I never made it into one myself). I think about all the passing through squeezed space I have done and am about to do, especially this next, drastic procedure, and wonder at the great, strange space in which I stand now, shafts of light falling on me at odd angles, aware of heaven above and the world around me and the other people: presaging a brave new world?

And we see you, E! Like a divine treat, a gentle, loving encounter to strengthen me.

We delight in Song Dong's (contemporary Chinese artist) clever, thought-provoking use of mirrors, doors, windows fastened and unfastened, intriguing objects and light fittings, photographs of basic human activity: eating, drinking, shitting, sleeping; three plates of food arranged like mountains with broccoli trees; Alice Through the Looking Glass. Preserving the old, mourning its loss, imprisoning beauty (China's lack of democracy?), doors opening on to what looks like another world but is just a mirror; daggers stabbing mandalas (China's treatment of Tibet?). Intriguing. He is as well known in China as Ai Weiwei.

I am hot. At a certain point, when no one is looking, I whip off my wig. I haven't brought a back-up hat, so this is another brave moment that, as soon as I have passed it, seems like nothing at all. Of course no one is looking at me. With my shaved head I look like quite a lot of people here in Burlington House. Another liberation.

Helene Schjerfbeck, Finnish, 1862–1946, celebrated as a master artist in Finland, is simply wonderful. There is a large room with all her self-portraits, begun when she was a child and ending just before she dies. Angular, bright, punky, ghostlike, perky, sharp-eyed, desperately sad, almost not there, stripped to her basic self, astonishing and true. I buy her catalogue and will take her into the Cotton Rooms with me. I think: I will take Giacometti too; I have his catalogue from the stupendous exhibition at the National Portrait Gallery from a while ago. I am absorbing art, Dear Readers, to take with me into my anchorhold; I feel as though I am bringing all humanity with me.

As we pass a random door wedge on a shelf, probably not an exhibit, Seán tells me, 'You are a Wedge: you wedge the door open for others to come through.' I am utterly delighted by this compliment. And later he says: 'You are my Wild Thing', quoting:

> I never saw a wild thing sorry for itself
> A small bird will drop frozen dead from a bough
> Without ever having felt sorry for itself.[2]

Again, I am utterly delighted, though I certainly AM sorry for myself sometimes.

You tell me, G, that you have designated a Gregorian chant as one through which you will commune with me. More special blessings flow. I would like to know which chant it is so I can listen too . . .

And that has given me this idea, a request to each of you, Dear Readers.

Would you tell me one piece of music that you love? It can be anything; it doesn't have to be holy or chosen with the thought that it will help me. What you love is what I want. I will create a playlist to take into my anchorhold and that way I will have the sound of your beloved souls with me as I journey through my treatment and recovery.

Friday, 18 October

A three-hour wait to see Dr Mary at the Guy's clinic is worth it when she tells me that my bone marrow biopsy shows that the myeloma has reduced to less than one per cent. When I was diagnosed in March it was ten to fifteen per cent. My kappa light chains, which came down from their dangerous 1,100 to twenty-four, if you remember, Dear Readers, after the first cycle of Carfilzomib, have stayed normal, and I have only two paraproteins left (no idea if I'm stating this in the technologically correct way). I am, says Dr Mary, in remission. I am in remission!!

So WHY am I about to have a stem cell transplant, killing all my bone marrow and rebooting my system so dramatically?

Because myeloma is incurable. Remission means just that: the myeloma has not gone altogether and it will come back sooner or later. The stem cell transplant is the best way to deepen the remission. So although I feel well, and the numbers say I am well, I am still going to go through with this.

But how confounding it is: I have to will my healthy body into painful, frightening, illness-inducing procedures and treatments.

Saturday, 19 October

Today the march for another Brexit referendum. Parliament will vote on whether to leave on 31 October. I said I would wear black if it is Brexit day, despite it also being my birthday. However, I now know I will be nearing the worst of the Melphalan marrow-death on that day: when my throat may feel as though it is coated in broken glass, when I shall be dripping diarrhoea, when I shall be at my lowest ebb, wanting to die, in a sense being very close to death like Julian. Is there now a chance that it won't be Brexit day after all? That would indeed be a mercy: one less thing to suffer.

Twenty-eighth Letter

Dear Readers

I wear my new tweed Peaky Blinders cap to mass but then on an impulse I bare my head for Fr Eamonn's blessing. He knows my story and confesses afterwards that my gesture brought tears to his eyes. As well as presenting my bared head to God, I am presenting Al the angel's gentle handiwork for a blessing too, a blessing that passes in my imagination to all the hurting Kurdish people.

We go for a long, tricky, muddy, hilly walk in Ecclesbourne Glen.

A day in UCLH. I have a kidney blood test, which involves being injected with a dye (more painful vein-hunting) at 10.14am (the exact time is noted) and returning at 12.14pm, 1.14pm and 2.14pm to have blood taken to see whether my kidneys have processed the dye (something like that).

Jackie, my clinical nurse specialist, kindly arranges my appointment with the consultant to fall in the first two-hour slot. Dr Neil is lovely, kind and straightforward. He has two disgustingly beautiful young medical students with him, one of whom irritates me further by unconsciously playing with her head of lustrous long hair when I speak about the trauma of losing mine. Actually, I'm not irritated by them at all, they are sweet and earnest, and wish me well with youthful enthusiasm when I leave. Dr Neil reminds me that myeloma is incurable. He is not impressed at my remission status: I still have the cancer and the stem cell transplant is the best chance of lengthening the remission, because the cancer will return at some point. He is not dismissive of the Cardamon trial, but he says that many other chemotherapies have been compared with stem cell transplant and nothing has been shown to better it yet. His confidence in the transplant does help me, I must say, let go of any lingering wish to be on the other arm of the study. It's just as well because we have to go through the side effects, including a two to three per cent chance of death, high likelihood of sore mouth (D's throat of broken glass, which I think 'sore' doesn't quite cover), fever, diarrhoea, nausea and fatigue. I will take three months to feel again as well as I do today.

I sign the consent form.

Thursday, 24 October

A blissful last pedicure with Elinor, who massages my feet tenderly and paints each of my toenails a different colour, a rainbow display of fiery orange and yellow and chestnut brown and red that will cheer me up in hospital. And then she gives me a facial with delicious smells I will soon not be able to bear, including an Indian head massage made much easier by my shorn head.

We have a last curry at the FILO (First In Last Out) pub and I muster the courage to remove my hat. Roy the waiter is a friend and knows we've been going through the mill, and is lovely. But then a hardly known neighbour trots up to our table and says, 'I had to come and speak to you. You look like a lady with a haircut she didn't want. What cancer have you got then?' I slowly unfreeze as it turns out this very day she has been recalled by the hospital because of a possible return of her own breast cancer, and is scared herself, but when she has gone all my brittle confidence in my bad-ass haircut has shattered, and I feel, again, exposed, vulnerable, an object of pity.

So it is not just with joy and laughter that I receive your poem, H, but deep gratitude too:

Your follicles may have lost their flossity
but you dear friend are alive with porosity
and though you're meeting your public less than hairily
you radiate loveliness ever more Claire-ily

And thank you, A, for telling me 'your qualities are far greater than you imagine' as I am still me, revealed under the hair.

Friday, 25 October

I have achieved a Laurence of Arabia look with your beautiful taupe scarf, H, under my riding hat, for my last ride this morning on Wooster, who behaves beautifully. The rain ceases just for the time we are out, and I soak up the sun and the view, the green and the turning leaves, the trees bending in the wind, the feeling of communion with Wooster as we move together, the gathering of my muscles and the strength of him, the strength of me. A leaf lands on my saddle and I put it carefully in my pocket, believing ever since I read Mary Poppins that it was lucky to catch an autumn leaf. As we arrive back, Chloe, who leads the ride and is among the kindest people I know, brings tears to my eyes as she says, 'Wooster always seems to know when he is needed.' I untack him and give him water and feel the warm breathing mass of him before we leave.

A consignment of logs arrives and we enjoy the satisfaction of stacking them, ready for when we are back and it is cold enough for a fire.

A final Pilates session with gentle instruction from Glenda about the exercises I can keep practising, no matter how weak I feel, over the next period.

I write a final email in an attempt to let the Institute go from my mind completely for a month.

Saturday, 26 October

We are ready to depart Hastings. The activities and tasks that lie between me and my transplant are completing themselves, and fear rises in me as I contemplate a return to London to face my destiny.

Seán says we should think of the next few weeks as going on a cruise. We will be in a cabin. Sometimes the weather will be stormy and there will be sea sickness and times of being confined to one's bed. Sometimes we will put in at a port and can venture out on dry land. There may be a breakout of listeria. It's a good metaphor, more deeply impressed upon me as we make one final pilgrimage to the sea's edge, standing on the harbour arm and watching, and being sprayed by, the immense, crashing, violent, boiling, energetic waves. I open myself to them as I have to the walks and rides and massages and art and conversations and your moving messages and music choices, all the wonderful things of these past two weeks. Interosculation and porosity. Communion. Non-separation. The universe in me as I enter my anchorhold, represented by my playlist, my leaf and a flat shell-like stone picked from the beach today.

Sunday, 27 October

In London, I practise cleaning my bottom with the shower. I am concerned about soreness and even the possibility of infection with diarrhoea which can be acidic and so painful for one's nether regions. Bidets are not luxuries: they are essential for cleanliness. But there are no bidets in the Cotton Rooms or the hospital. My perch on the edge of the bath is possible now, while I am energetic and healthy and strong, but I still manage to spray water all over the bathroom as well as myself. It will be impossible if I am weak. But having a full body shower every time one visits the lavatory, which will be a frequent occurrence, seems ridiculous, especially as one will need to moisturise afterwards as well.

Note my lapse into the coy 'one'. These are intimate problems.

It takes me all morning to pack. I will be in the Cotton Rooms and need outdoor clothes to walk to the Cancer Centre each day; I will almost certainly end up in an isolation room in UCLH and need changes of nightclothes and comfortable kaftan-like day clothes. I want to look good and I think hard about colours — I have a lot of differently hued hats now — as well as comfort and practicality. Dear H, both your scarves will be a blessing and much used, as will yours, J.

I take as long deciding what to bring to feed my inner self. The Dear Readers' playlist. Julian of course, and the Bible, and your book with Philippa, N, on the religious life, and Simon's book on prayer; also Antony Gormley's book on sculpture. I have Helen Schjerfbeck's catalogue, and Giacometti's, but they are both so heavy and I already have so much to take. But I think they will be good to look at when I can't think, when I am at my lowest, while I am listening to your music. I have paper to write on, and paper to paint on, and paints. I have a Pilates theraband and your 'Hastings series' of cards, J, which I will place on the windowsills to cheer me up.

I am finally done at lunchtime and meet Seán for a long stroll in Kew Gardens, a final breath of green, turning trees, the magnificent glass houses, a little Chihuly glass sculpture, a cup of tea . . . oh dear, what a tedious account of not very much, but it is precious to me, Dear Readers.

I return to the flat and the clang of the gate closing sounds portentous.

I suddenly remember that tomorrow, the day I receive the killer Melphalan, is the fifteenth anniversary of my father's death from cancer. I feel I am joining him, sort of.

I wonder if I can have my stem cells blessed before they are given back to me?

Oh, I am scared.

I am strong.

See you on the other side.

The following diary entries are written up from scrawled notes while I was in hospital. I was too ill to type and only sent a brief message when I could to my Dear Readers, who received the following pages in December, when I could bear to look back at what I had been through.

Twenty-ninth Letter

Dear Readers

I walk towards my fear.

Today is the fifteenth anniversary of my father's death from cancer and it is the day of my own little death from Melphalan, the chemo-therapy that will kill my bone marrow. It is based on the mustard gas used in the First World War.

The taxi driver takes a complex route, distracting me with side streets I'd not seen before. It is 8.00am when we arrive, so I take my luggage to the Cotton Rooms: an embarrassingly vast case, packed with day clothes and night clothes in anticipation of weeks away, and a lot of books.

And I walk empty handed to the Cancer Centre, to 'ambulatory care' – where the Cotton Room patients and other outpatients are treated. I see the registrar, who tells me I will feel all right for the next couple of days. He is beautiful.

I am sent to the basement to have my PICC line inserted. 'PICC' stands for 'peripherally inserted central catheter'. The nurse-surgeon is beautifully made up under her face visor. She runs a very fine tube into a vein through my upper left arm, all the way to the other side of my heart. She is in training, so I get to hear the explanation and directions of the senior nurse, and watch, fascinated, a living cross section of my pumping vein on the screen as the line is fed through it. Afterwards two exit valves dangle from my arm so blood can be taken and substances infused without having to puncture my skin and damage my veins with cannulas every time. A clever invention, great not to have cannulas, and I can't feel it, but it is strange to have inside me. I don't like it.

I meet M, a fellow myeloma sufferer. M's myeloma is 'galloping' and this is his second stem cell transplant after only ten weeks since his first. Ten weeks! He lives in Broadstairs and is a magician. He wears a pork pie hat and answers all my questions about the procedure kindly and reassuringly, but his eyes are scared: he knows what is coming.

Then I meet the consultant, Dr Neil. Because I have compromised kidney function my body won't tolerate the Melphalan so well (but what would 'tolerating it well' look like?) and the issue for me, he says, will be nausea. Straightaway, not in two days. Cold dread seizes me.

We have until 2.30pm. Seán has arrived and we check in to the Cotton Rooms. We choose a quiet room looking over the back of the Cancer Centre, not such an interesting view but Tottenham Court Road is noisy. I don't know how long we will be here. It is lovely to have the comfort of a room we can share. But as soon as my temperature goes up to thirty-eight degrees I have to go into hospital because it means I have an infection, and since this happens to ninety-five per cent of people having a stem cell transplant it is likely to happen to me. Once the Melphalan has killed off the bone marrow I am neutropenic, with no immunity at all. Even bacteria in my own body which I would normally tolerate can cause infection, and infection will kill if not treated.

But I feel a challenge: I want to be one of the five per cent who don't have to leave the comfort of the Cotton Rooms during the whole procedure.

I return to ambulatory care for the Melphalan. I sit in one of the squishy chemotherapy chairs, just like those at Guy's but in sicklier colours. Nurse Lydia solemnly hands me a tray of five orange-flavoured popsicles and I'm told to start sucking them. This is to counter the Melphalan side effect of destroying the bacteria lining my digestive system from my mouth all the way down to my bottom. I am hooked up to the drip and given a flush of saline, then the Melphalan starts. I sit and suck as the Melphalan infuses. I look and feel ridiculous, which makes me laugh, even as I receive the poison.

It only takes half an hour, but it is a killer. I suck my popsicles and meditate on *maranatha*.

Then it is finished and we are free to go. I am given three kinds of anti-emetic as well as stomach protector, anti-viral drugs and vitamin D3 for my bones. A huge bag of drugs.

I feel strange. I have some mouth ulcers (already) and a slightly queasy stomach.

I do gentle Pilates and my head stops feeling like cotton wool.

I do not feel sick. I do not feel sick.

We spend the evening in our room, Seán on the phone for a long time to neighbours in Hastings because our house alarm has gone off.

Tuesday, 29 October

I have hardly slept and feel shivery, queasy, sniffly. It occurs to me that the one thing that cannot happen now is that I do not receive my stem cell transplant, scheduled for tomorrow. I have had the killer Melphalan; if I don't have my stem cells I will die.

I throw up.

I am in a kind of anticipatory Easter — today is anticipatory Saturday, yesterday was Good Friday, tomorrow will be my resurrection; only the effects are all delayed so my actual Easter Saturday will start at the weekend when my bone marrow dies and who knows when resurrection will dawn with the stem cells grafting?

I am wondering what happens to the dead bone marrow. Is it absorbed into the bone 'wall' surrounding it? Like humus from dead leaves into the ground?

Over the day I eat a little cheese and biscuits, stale pain au raisin, wafer biscuits, bean salad, cornflakes . . . I didn't realise when Dr Neil said 'Nausea will be an issue for you' he meant it will be an issue because I will lose my appetite and stop eating before I *really* lose my appetite when the Melphalan starts killing my bone marrow. I can't lose strength now. So I eat exactly what I fancy, when I fancy it.

A feeling of positivity and well-being rises in me, despite how odd I feel physically. A positive attitude makes the stem cell transplant work, said the nurse who gave me the popsicles.

I won't be sick. I won't.

I am.

It is such a relief to be sick because it takes the nausea away, but it also takes away the banana I have just eaten, with great difficulty, and all the drugs I have just swallowed through my sore and swelling throat.

Everyone in the Cotton Rooms is sensitive to each other's need to be apart and careful, as well as sociable. Only one too-hearty greeting and interrogation, but they are couched in kindness and love.

I return to ambulatory care for my stem cell transplant. I am in a separate room, on a bed. I am cannulated for this; for some reason the PICC line won't do. Nurse Lydia brings in two frozen bags of what looks like gloopy blood, the stem cells I last saw hooked up to Rosie. She thaws them in a bath of warm water in the room. First one, then the other bag is infused into me. It is straightforward apart from the moment when the stem cells congregate in the vein around the cannula and get stuck, and Lydia has to push them onwards and into my body with a flush. That hurts a lot. I lie and listen to my Dear Reader playlist, which brings me joy. The procedure takes about two hours.

At the end, one of the hospital chaplains appears and gives me Communion. We are left alone for the little service, which is inexpressibly comforting, even though she drops things and emphasises the word 'hope' in a pleading, needy way that would normally have irritated me. Now I am simply grateful and tearful. My blood pressure has come right down, having been high after the transplant. Lydia says it is because I have had Communion. She wears a tiny gold cross on a necklace.

I am overcome with emotion.

I vomit during the night.

It is my birthday.

A huge card lit by fairy lights from Seán in the worst possible taste makes me laugh. He gives me a horse shoe for my birthday present.

We stroll slowly to Gordon Square and Woburn Square and relish the trees, their leaves turning orange and tawny and yellow and old gold.

I manage to eat some yoghurt and some stale croissant, a pear and some biscuits and cheese.

I am very low. The thought of going back to the Cancer Centre and being among the drips and the chemotherapy and the needles and the calm, accepting patients fills me with dread and nausea.

I don't ask for prayers to change the course of history but oh, dear Lord, I pray that this cup is taken from me soon, and that I go into such a deep remission that I never have to cross the threshold of any cancer centre ever again.

I feel sick, tired, dopey, sad, useless, bloated, hot, and the Melphalan side effects, apart from nausea, haven't even begun yet.

I will forget how bad this is once it is over; a mercy perhaps but I never want to have to go through it again.

Oh Julian, you fixed your mind on God and you were not troubled by earthly things. Help me to be the same. Help me.

I realise, as I cry and pace the room, that I *can* ask you, my Dear Readers, for help. This is strange and hard: I don't like asking for myself and I am unable to imagine an interventionist God. But I remember how I prayed so desperately and sincerely for Seán's health to be restored and feel I can, this time, ask for myself.

I write to you a single line of email: Pray for me!

Friday, 1 November

A flood of messages from you: 'I am on my knees now'; 'I'm praying like crazy and I don't have a god to pray to'; 'I dedicate to you all the energy and strength of my yoga practice'. And the deeply reassuring responses from those of you who have practised a lifetime of prayer. Your prayers in all their forms are a benison. How amazing you are, how grateful I am.

And I feel better today. It won't last – I still have to go through the neutropenic stage when my bone marrow dies – but for now, today, I have some strength. You have led me to the deep inner peace that the world cannot give.

Saturday, 2 November

I take an age to swallow my supper of pale cheese and biscuits and yoghurt. Every mouthful is a struggle. I have no appetite whatsoever; my throat is swollen; my mouth is sticky with mucous. But I manage some food ('don't get out of the habit of eating', says the registrar).

Then I vomit, copiously. It feels as though a hard day's work has been destroyed.

But the will to live is in me.

Sunday, 3 November

I have diarrhoea. I sweat in the night. I have a red, angry, itchy rash all over my neck and torso. I imagine the Melphalan as an evil creature, thinking up additional tortures to test my endurance and my tolerance to their limit. I feel like Job.

The thought of opening my laptop brings its own particular queasiness to my stomach, but it is Sunday and I want to keep faith with you, Dear Readers. I manage to write this: 'There is no letter this week, just a heartfelt thank you, from my place of weakness, for your prayers.'

Monday, 4 November

I am subject to double sneezes that come out in hysterical splurts. My throat is swollen. I am nauseous, nauseous, nauseous. And now, diarrhoea. I can't just lie in bed and quietly die. I have my daily challenges: I must eat and keep the food I manage to swallow down. I must take my drugs, drink as much water as I can, get up, shower, dress, walk to the Cancer Centre. If I do these things, it is enough. I am exhausted and rest between every action.

When I rest, semi-comatose, not sleeping, I meditate on *maranatha*. I cannot think or make sense of anything, but I can repeat my mantra like a golden thread.

I have diarrhoea, which means I might have an infection, so I am put in an isolation room in ambulatory care when I visit today. Seán and I gently sing Robert Stone's 'Our Father'. I find a deep peace at the heart of my weakness. I am helplessly spinning through the universe, subject to forces I know not of. There is nothing I can do. I am relaxed.

But trying not to vomit brings me back to the vile reality of my physical state. I have to attend to my body: eat, drink, take drugs, not throw up.

Tuesday, 5 November

Seán is really and truly a saint. I have to produce a diarrhoea sample and I cannot look at any of my bodily excretions without involuntarily producing more of them. Seán collects the sample for me from the collecting thing I evacuate into. I evacuate and immediately leave the bathroom, blessing Seán with all my heart; but I can't avoid seeing from the corner of my eye that what I have produced is bright, chemical yellow. Mustard gas!

I am dragging my body through the week, moving like a snail through the world. I feel worse and worse. This is day six from the transplant; Dr Neil says these are the worst days. I breathe: it is enough. I swallow a little food: it is enough. I don't throw it up again: it is enough.

I manage one quarter of a tuna sandwich. It is a perfectly good, simple sandwich, but in my mouth it is dry and almost impossible to chew and swallow.

I cannot clean my teeth. My mouth is full of ulcers, my tongue is coated in slime, my throat is swollen, everything hurts; and worst of all even putting the soft-brushed toothbrush my lovely hygienist gave me for just this eventuality into my mouth produces a gagging reaction and I throw up. I have a mouthwash: that will have to be enough for now.

I am cold. I am dead to the world we pass through on our way to the Cancer Centre. I am in Easter Saturday.

The nurse tells me I am neutropenic. That means my immune system has gone completely.

Wednesday, 6 November

My temperature has risen to 37.8 degrees.

I am given a plasma transplant. Thank you, anonymous A+ blood donor.

I didn't want to be admitted but I am so weak and nauseous that when, at 8.00pm this evening, my temperature is thirty-eight degrees and I have to ring the helpline and am told to come in, I am relieved. We walk slowly to the main hospital and I am put in Room 6 of Ward 13 North. Seán returns to the Cotton Rooms: he will check out tomorrow, and go home.

I vomit.

Overnight my blood pressure, oxygen level and temperature are checked every four hours. I am given an antibiotic infusion for the infection every six hours. Blood is taken and tested. Nurses come in and out and do things to me as I lie helplessly being kept alive.

Thursday, 7 November

I receive a visit: 'I'm A, the ward administrator.' A sort of leaps about the room in discomfort, not looking at me. He gives me a letter which tells me that when I am discharged I must leave quickly and quietly. Things would run so much more smoothly if it weren't for you patients, his body language tells me.

Everything is taken out of my hands. Drugs administered. Attached to a drip for antibiotics and anything else I need. Blood taken. I don't have to think about anything except what to ask for for meals, which is hard enough. I sleep fitfully between the interruptions that keep me alive. Blessed Seán arrives with a fresh nightshirt to replace the one drenched in my sweat, parcels and post from the flat, the *Evening Standard*, sanity and his quiet, calming attention.

Friday, 8 November

The Horror. The Horror. How can anyone feel like this and keep on being alive and human? Next door a man is shouting and I cannot imagine where he finds the energy.

The cruelty of Melphalan, destroying my alimentary canal when I need it so badly to get well again. Nausea and diarrhoea; nausea and diarrhoea. I cannot clean my teeth. I sweat. My bathroom is cold and the shower, which I force myself to use every day, is a mean dribble, leaving me in tears and nauseated because I am so cold. But I must moisturise my shivering, scaly, skinny body before I put my nightshirt back on.

I am in hell, being tortured.

But hell is a bright, clean room, and my torturers, the nurses, healthcare assistants, cleaning staff, the beautiful man who takes my reluctant food orders, are all full of kindness.

I listen to my Dear Readers' playlist. It is on shuffle as I am absolutely incapable of making choices. But the right music plays: Finzi's 'Life is a flower in springtime'; Mozart's *Requiem* with his commanding 'light perpetual shine on you'; Leonard Cohen's 'You want it darker (I'm ready, Lord)'. The music sings in my soul, rallying my spirit, accompanying and articulating my pain and confusion and utter vulnerability when I have no resources of my own, nothing.

Sometimes I feel I am in a place of helpless deep peace. And right at the heart of that helplessness: the will to live.

I am a pupa in my cocoon of Room 6. What lies beyond the door tempts me not one jot. The view from the window – magnificent, as I am on the thirteenth floor and can see a long way north – is of another world not my own.

I need proper chicken soup from my Jewish relatives. Beloved S, you understand when I phone you and cry and ask if you would make me some.

Saturday, 9 November

Nurse Francis tells me I will feel worse before I feel better. What?! How long can a body endure what I have endured? How much more pain can I take? But then he realises I am on day nine from my transplant, not day two as he had thought, and corrects his prediction. I should be coming out of my neutropenic phase. I want to hit him and hug him at the same time. But I'm hooked up to a fucking drip of some substance or other and can do neither.

I think of Julian and how she ignored the pain of her illness, concentrating on Christ whom she loved so much. How different I am, lost horrendously in my bodily suffering, not a vision of Jesus in sight. But even Julian cries out for her pain to stop when she experiences in her own body Christ's pains as he is dying on the cross. She says his (and her) terrible pain continued as his dying stretched out, as it seemed, for a 'sennyght'. My own suffering is so stretched out, getting much worse when I think it can't get any worse, on and on for days and days and days. And now I feel I am not alone, and I am comforted.

Beloved S, you bring me the chicken soup and I am able to drink some. I am convinced it helps. I keep it down.

And then my temperature spikes to thirty-eight degrees in the night.

Sunday, 10 November

At the 4.15am check up I am no longer neutropenic, the nurse tells me. My stem cells are up and at it and I'm out the other side. Except that I'm not. I hurt all over. Bone pain from the stem cells, my throat hurts, I have a temperature, I have diarrhoea and I'm crying my eyes out.

My hair has not completely fallen out. It has moulted so my pink scalp is visible through Al's beautiful shriven hair, but it's my old hair. I am so glad I cut it all off though. D was right: it really is the last thing to be worrying about when every other part of my body is suffering. At least moulting doesn't hurt. Isn't it ironic that hair loss was my biggest fear? It is nothing, nothing, compared to the rest of my woes.

I manage an email to you: 'I am crawling out of hell. But the doctors say my case is "plain sailing". I shudder for those of my fellow patients who did not sail well. I should be home mid-week.'

Monday, 11 November

Life is quickening within me. The icon of the 'harrowing of hell' gives me an image to rest with, thank you, M: I picture Jesus grasping my wrist firmly to bring me crawling out of the worst time in my life.

And Vaughan Williams' 'Lark Ascending' from you, dear A, plays at the exact right moment, and I weep again, copiously, this time for the sweet, delicate, fierce and unstoppable force of life the violin expresses, that I feel in me.

Like Lazarus I am casting off my grave clothes. It is strenuous, an effort I mostly don't want, at all, to make. I want to stay cocooned, sleeping, but now that I'm no longer neutropenic I should exercise. I pull on my clothes (my grave clothes? They are the ones I arrived in and they are now too big for me), and go for a tiny walk, hanging on to Seán. The effort it takes is phenomenal: slowly, slowly walking to the lift, slowly through the crowded foyer, slowly out into strange air I have not breathed since I 'died', and just a few steps outside, to the corner of the building, not on busy Euston Road but at the quieter back entrance. And mysteriously Life — I don't know what else to call it — comes to meet my hard work: I feel a quickening response that is as much from outside as it is from within me.

You come and give me Holy Communion and the sacrament for the sick, dear M. You don't drop anything, and you have dignity of bearing and voice, and you create a holy place in sterile Room 6 with the sacred ritual. I am infected by holiness! Thank you.

Tuesday, 12 November

I want to go home and the consultant has said, all being well, I can . . . but my temperature keeps spiking. If I went home and my temperature reached thirty-eight degrees I would have to go to A & E so there is no way that I will be allowed home while this is happening.

My windows are cleaned today by a young man who could have been cleaning anyone's windows, but here he is in my sterile box. It feels surreal, like two worlds colliding.

I do a little Pilates; Seán takes me for a slightly longer walk. I make myself eat though I have absolutely no appetite. I want to go home.

Wednesday, 13 November

My temperature has gone up to 38.6. I do feel ill. I swallow paracetamol which brings the temperature down but then it goes up again. I
am not such a straightforward case after all, and I won't be going
home for a while. But inside myself I feel a deeper will than my own
stirring, and I hear the same deep will stirring in Brahms' *Requiem*:
thank you, T. I eat, do Pilates, walk a little further outside with Seán.

Friday, 15 November

Am I still going through death? Or am I in the womb, waiting to be
born? Am I Theseus, finding my way out of the labyrinth, my mantra
perhaps my thread to guide me? Or am I Jonah, cast into the vasty
deep, swimming upwards towards the light and the breathable air?

I am mostly failing to clean my teeth because it still makes me gag.
I worry about them. I have to drink pints of water and I cannot
abide the taste without some lemon cordial added: sugar constantly
coating my teeth, only a mouthwash to counter the rot.

Saturday, 16 November

I bark with laughter as the playlist shuffles to Alanis Morissette's
'Thank you' (thank you, K). The first line is 'How about getting off
these antibiotics?' Because my temperature won't stabilise, I have a
chest CT scan which shows a slight change not inconsistent with a
fungal infection. So now I am receiving a generic antibiotic *and* an
anti-fungal antibiotic called (something like) Caspar.

My PICC line has been removed, in case it was a cause of infection (it wasn't) so I'm being repeatedly, painfully cannulated again,
on top of daily puncturing for blood tests. Every morning at breakfast time a cheery phlebotomist comes and takes blood from me. I
hate them for sticking yet another needle in me; I love them for
being so jolly and kind. The cannulas are another thing altogether.
Every vein is sore and suffering. Even really competent, experienced
nurses struggle to find one that can take a cannula and the infusion
it brings. Seán and I sing the Stone 'Our Father' as the nurse wiggles

the needle into the vein, poking and exploring, hurting me dreadfully but necessarily. No cannula lasts more than two infusions before becoming so sore it has to be removed. I take as many drugs as I can by mouth. My body shrinks from invasion. How long, oh Lord, how long must I endure?

I am still nauseous. In the night a nurse approaches me like Sister Gilchrist in Alan Bennett's *Allelujah* brandishing an injection of an anti-emetic. 'Go away!' I say. 'No more needles.' She is not pleased. Soon she reappears to tell me I have to have my blood cultures taken. It feels like a punishment. It is 2.00am: why do I have to give blood cultures at 2.00am? I weep bitter tears as another gentle, lovely nurse takes the blood.

I have had enough.

Sunday, 17 November

I have to provide a sample of my diarrhoea. Ali, my healthcare assistant, has to collect the obediently filled receptacle as I cannot go near it. She tells me that the people who test stool samples at UCLH receive thousands of them a day. Imagine. Imagine a laboratory receiving all that poo.

We go for a walk and for the first time I feel the outside world is my home, not Room 6.

Today I manage to write to you: 'You have asked about visiting, which is really kind. I'm not seeing visitors at the moment as I'm still like a wounded animal (actually more like a shrivelled pixie) curled up in her corner and hurting. But you are all in this room with me already . . . And from the depths of my heart, thank you, I, for this quotation from Julian that landed in my inbox at exactly the right moment: "He said not 'Thou shalt not be tempested, thou shalt not be travailed, thou shalt not be dis-eased'; but he said, 'Thou shalt not be overcome'".'

Monday, 18 November

I am low on fluids and the infusions to top me up last eight hours. EIGHT hours attached to a drip. I have to have two of them. I submit with little grace, but the prospect of eight hours' imprisonment produces a kind of 'fuck it' energy to get dressed and go out with Seán for some fresh air first. The doctor says my 'fuck it' is evidence that I am getting better.

Tuesday, 19 November

I am enjoying listening to the Radio 4 series of reflections on George Eliot through her characters, fascinated to hear the suggestion that Eliot identified with Dorothea (in *Middlemarch*), as she sought an older man as her life partner because she wanted to follow intellectual pursuits rather than babies and things; but also that Eliot identified with Casaubon, the grim older man whom Dorothea married, who had dedicated his life to writing a definitive account of mythology that was obsolete long before he had finished writing it, and lived in dread of finding his life's work amounted to nothing (which it did). Eliot too feared that her books would have no future. I identify with her urges and fears.

Wednesday, 20 November

The nurses are superstars. Their shifts are twelve-and-a-half hours long, with a handover at 7.30am and 7.30pm. Each morning and each evening my nurse for the day comes and introduces herself. She (usually a she) has four patients to keep alive on this ward of twenty-four patients. The healthcare assistants, also stars, change my bed each day and answer when I press the buzzer, while the nurses are more technical and medical: they give me pills; cannulate me; hook me up to drips of fluid, antibiotic, magnesium, potassium, whatever, when I need them. I tell them I feel sick: they give me anti-emetic drugs. I have a temperature: they give me paracetamol. They are in and out of my room efficiently and quickly. But the manner of the giving of drugs and the poking of needles is delightful, for the most part, and all the care comes from love. And when I weep, or laugh, or express my frustration, they stop, and listen; sit down; hold my hand. Ru and Gill are ace cannulators though even their skills are tested by my rebellious veins. Ru is from the Philippines where she trained. Philippine-trained nurses arrive with all the necessary skills; British-trained nurses have to learn to cannulate and take blood once they arrive on the ward; these hands-on skills are deemed too danger-ous to be taught to trainees. They used to learn by practising on each other, Evelyn tells me. Now they learn on patients: she cannulates me under the supervision of a more senior nurse. She does well but the cannula lasts only for one infusion and is then too sore to be used again.

Whose bright idea was it to withdraw the bursary for a nurse's training? There are 40,000 unfilled training places. Why would you incur thousands of pounds in debt to be trained for a badly paid job?

Today I have a sweet, newly trained nurse, anxiously ensuring that everything she does, and I do, is correct. I love her but she is driving me MAD.

I am weighed. Before the transplant I was sixty-nine kilograms. I am sixty-two now. That's not all that light; in fact it's about the right weight for my height, but I am, I assure you, a shrivelled pixie.

Thursday, 21 November

I have started lying about my symptoms. I deny I have any because every time I name one I receive a drug to deal with it. I am in wholehearted rebellion against being treated like a machine.

Friday, 22 November

Today I am able to walk on Seán's arm all the way to Gordon Square, which has become a holy destination. We can stroll under the trees away from the traffic, weakly shuffle the fallen autumn leaves and sit and receive nature's generous healing touch. Under normal circum-stances it would take five minutes to walk there but to me it is a marathon. The trees are golden, the grass is green. We eat cake from Ginger Jules' café and drink coffee, sitting in the damp autumnal square. I am breathing, relearning how to live as a human being in the outside air. It feels miraculous. I take nothing for granted. One tawny leaf on the ground by my foot is pure, living joy, incorrigible, unstoppable, regardless of my state of being. Joy bubbles up and offers herself, and I say yes.

Saturday, 23 November

Nurse Anzie takes my temperature and it is 36.5. I start to believe that one day I will be home again. The CT scan has been rechecked and declared free of fungal infection, so I am off Caspar. My other antibiotic can be taken orally. No more infusions! No more cannulas!

Sunday, 24 November

And, all of a sudden, a message from the doctors: 'The lady in Room 6 can be discharged.' What is the word for relief when it is relief times a hundred? I write and tell you just this: 'I am going home.'

Monday, 25 November

I sweat dreadfully in the night but my temperature does not go up. I am home. Home!

Tuesday, 26 November

I eat a boiled egg. Despite the vile taste that lingers on my tongue like a dry paste, I can taste the egg and I relish it.

And I have some acupuncture from our dear friend Weidong. I feel my weakness and he is very gentle and careful. I weep.

Thursday, 28 November

Emerging from the flat for our daily constitutional, we discover a lunchtime concert at St George the Martyr and I listen, entranced, to a beautiful young pianist from Portugal play Bach, Mendelssohn and Debussy. Then we slowly stroll down Tabard Street and have coffee in the bar of the little Kino in Bermondsey Square. Up Bermondsey Street to London Bridge and Snowsfields, my stomach lurching as we approach Guy's. A good long walk. Back to the flat triumphant, clutching the *Evening Standard*.

Friday, 29 November

Eastwards along the Thames on her south bank, all the way to Butler's Wharf. Fresh clear air fills my lungs as we pass the ubiquitous German Christmas market wooden huts outside Hays Galleria, and stop at City Hall to watch the children running, shrieking and laughing, through the dancing water that fountains up out of the ground in unpredictable bursts. Bridge Theatre sheds warm light through its big glass doors. Returning inland along Tooley Street, we walk straight into the terror of the London Bridge tragedy. Fear ignites and spreads as people are suddenly running towards us, away from the Bridge, but we are commanded and comforted by tannoy to come into the station away from danger. I am struck, even in this moment, by how tender the announcement sounds. The running in visceral fear stops and people are quiet and responsible, not inflaming a volatile situation. They are on their phones, stories passing back and forth: 'There were shots'; 'It's more than one incident'; 'Borough Market is being evacuated'; 'Several people are dead' . . . We pass into and through London Bridge station to Newcomen Street and home.

Sunday, 1 December

This is my day: I wake up, have a cup of tea, rest, have a second cup of tea, eat some pear and yoghurt, rest, totter upstairs for some porridge, rest, shower, rest, clean my teeth (at last I can though they are sensitive), rest, dress, rest, apply make up, rest, go for a walk, rest . . . It takes all day just to do the things one needs to do to stay alive.

I write you a note: 'My heartfelt thanks for your terrible jokes (particularly appropriate, A, thank you: "What's brown and sticky? A stick") and for your gifts and letters and emails and your silent attention. I love them all and am supported by them; I am so helpless myself.'

I suck in my belly button as directed by Pilates and wince at the wrinkly thing my tummy has become. The dangers of losing weight when one is older!

I go to Guy's for blood tests. Later the haematology nurse phones to say my calcium is raised. I am instructed to stop taking the calcium tablets (hurray!) and to return for more blood tests on Friday to check that has worked. Anything, anything at all if it means no readmission to hospital. No temperature spikes but my blood pressure is low – a hundred over something. No wonder I feel weak.

More acupuncture and I realise how much strength I have gained just in one week.

I don my wig. It was to have been a gear change, a step up towards recovery, but I think I look alien: the wig which is so like the hair I had before Al shrove me is no longer who I am. I feel inauthentic. I'm a shrivelled pixie now, not the woman I was.

Our walks are longer every day: today we reach the Garden Museum by Lambeth Palace. The museum is a charming creation, fitting neatly within the original St Mary's church without detracting from the building, which you can still appreciate – like the clever and sensitive new refectory Stephen Platten built within the original medieval monks' refectory at Norwich Cathedral. Thirsty for nature, we have been seeking out parks in all our walks, and finding them, thanks mainly to Southwark Council, in the most unlikely corners. The museum gives context and meaning to parks and gardening and the human relationship with nature that they embody.

Thursday, 5 December

At last I open my laptop and begin to write up what has happened to me from my scribbled notes, jotted down even on the worst days so that I would have a record. I feel strong enough to look back at them and let them rekindle my memory so that I can describe them. I shy away from the trauma but I want to keep on telling it as honestly and clearly as I can. I began writing to you because I wanted to tell the whole story, including the best and the worst, most visceral, revolting human physical side of it, as well as the extraordinary transcendent joy of it. But I particularly want to describe the physical reality of the transplant because I do not think that any human being should give another human being Melphalan. We cancer patients cannot refuse Melphalan: what choice do we have? But if the medics can really hear how appalling, brutal and inhumane a treatment it is, is there a chance the research question will be asked: is there an alternative to Melphalan for stem cell transplant?

Saturday, 7 December

I do what is needed to keep on the journey to full health but find I have little inner resource: my characteristic psychological positivity has all but deserted me. I am not depressed, not at all, but I am passive. I haven't the strength to pull myself up by my own bootstraps.

But I am at last strong enough to read a poem. This one, thank you, dear S, speaks loudly to my state, and I love it because it beautifully mirrors Seán's own experience as a four-year-old in Knockanure:

> Alerted in the hayfield by a shout
> I catch the small grey thing
> that scuttles from my scythe and me
> and yield it to the keeping of Fiona
> who is three.
> You could blow it out this thing,
> it is so small and weak;
> it is a tail dependent on a squeak,
> a palpitation trimmed with fur.

Fiona has no words for it, no thought even,
she has narrowed down in being
to a pair of childish hands
and yet the weakness she is learning now
will stay with her
through all her lives and all her lands
until its turn comes round again.
Unrecognised, perhaps unwanted then,
the meaning of this day
will flood out over husband, lover, child, whoever
has the good luck to have chanced upon her
and to be standing in her way.[4]

I have been — still am — that field mouse in Fiona's hands, my life utterly dependent upon her will to keep me alive, able to do nothing for myself.

What is the point of utter weakness? What purpose does it serve? What can it do or achieve? What glory is there in it? What is there to respect in it? Believe in it? Offer reasons for following it? None. Absolutely none. And yet look what the field mouse gave Fiona.

Thirtieth Letter

Dear Readers

I read a piece in *The Oldie* by William Cook about taking Auberon Waugh's advice to be kind, rather than right: Cook was amazed to find, having been brought up staunchly socialist, that most Conservatives he got to know were nicer than he was. He noticed that right-wing papers were much better at paying his fees than left-wing ones. I am reminded of a piece of advice handed down to me by Robin Lorrimer, Balliol man from a previous generation: 'Drink with the Right, vote with the Left.'

Cook in turn offers excellent advice: actively seek out kind people, whether or not you agree with them. You'll have a good eclectic and intellectually stimulating group of friends / work colleagues. Auberon Waugh deliberately wrote for the *New Statesman* despite being of a different political hue; Cook wrote for the *Mail* and the *Telegraph*, and not, I think, just because they paid on time. It's delightful and educational, being with people who disagree with you, if they're kind. I realise that you, Dear Readers, are a community of kindness. You do not all agree with my views, religious, political, social or philosophical, but you are never less than kind.

I have difficult nights and where is God then? I toss and turn and sweat and feel abandoned. Today, I feel suffused with love and my head bows as I receive what feels like a blessing suddenly. Why now, though? Why not in the night, when I feel so much in need of comfort?

Lord Byron's poem, J, arrives from you in the midst of my

thoughts. You say it is 'For Claire, when she is sleeping'. Byron writes of the joy felt by those who 'watch o'er what they love while sleeping', and the tranquility of the one who sleeps: 'stirless, helpless, and unmoved'.[5] *There* is God in the night. Watching with you, J, and other J who told me last May to sleep and leave the praying to the Dear Readers. And then you, a third J, write: 'They that wait upon the Lord shall renew their strength'(Isaiah 40:31, KJV). Three Js, all magnifying my blessing. Thank you.

I want my hair back now. With all the moulting I look like a tufty fledgling. Seán massages my head with olive oil to stimulate the follicles. Will I grow some new hair?? Now my scalp is shiny and reflects in the light between the lonely shafts of single silvery hairs.

Thursday, 12 December

My hair's recovery is slower than the rest of me. As I gain strength, I look for its responding length. Alas, I am still a tufty fledgling, my olive oiled and massaged scalp under one of those hotel shower caps, looking ridiculous. Lolling in bed, to let the olive oil seep into my scalp before showering.

I vote tactically but, standing in the polling booth with my pencil hovering, it feels like a betrayal. From the very first time I voted, that moment in the little private space created by the then sweetly makeshift wooden-with-crumpled-green-cotton-curtain-for-privacy booth, now rather nasty-lightweight-plastic-like-a-cheap-toy booth, one voter directly confronting a group of potential leaders and choosing one of them, the experience has had a kind of holy aura for me. Representative democracy at work. A citizen granted the right to choose her political leaders. Aren't we fortunate?

(Which is why the EU referendum felt so wrong. One human being, not a representative politician, making the most preposterously enormous choice that should not have been mine to make, but that of those who wittingly shoulder the burden of government. It was like being asked to conduct life-changing surgery without any training. Wearing a blindfold.)

Friday, 13 December

Oh dear.

Sunday, 15 December

I wonder what it is all for.

And I choose: this new life granted to me shall be lived in praise of God and service of humanity and the planet. A rededication. I don't know what I mean by either of my dedications, but I want to learn.

Dear Readers, I am much, much better. The stem cell transplant is fading into the past. Thank heavens for being left alone (mostly) by hospitals, being allowed to recover, to gain strength not just physically but psychologically. Dear Lord, please let this hard-won new life not be in vain.

Thirty-first Letter

Dear Readers

Monday, 16 December

I feel like a scab that is drying and about to fall off. Scratchy and irritable, alive and itching to feel the air on my skin.

Thursday, 19 December

It is day fifty since my transplant and I have a meeting with one of the haematology registrars at UCLH for the halfway-to-recovery check up. I am doing well on all fronts. He cannot say when this horrible taste in my mouth will finally depart, but it will gradually reduce as my energy gradually increases. Nurse Zoe says I will have some new hair starting to grow in about two weeks' time. Curly baby hair alongside my thin but still-growing dead straight crew cut.

I make my point about the need to find an alternative to Melphalan and the doctor says that he hears me. I discover today that I had the highest possible dose of the nasty stuff, but he and Zoe acknowledge that my concerns are not based on my having had a worse experience than most, because I didn't. My case, until the late onset of additional infection, which was frustrating rather than painful, was 'plain sailing'. But the motivation to generate research questions which seek to replace Melphalan with something less toxic and torturing will only arise if the medics hear the pain of their patients. I ask the registrar to listen (not talk) to the nurses who keep us alive once the Melphalan starts its nasty work: they see the suffering close up.

A keen person in reception hands me a questionnaire about my experience of UCLH. How likely am I to recommend UCLH to others?

Why, oh *why*, do governments think the public wants CHOICE in relation to our healthcare? How can a market mindset improve things? All it does is make me worry: Is my doctor worse than others? If I am ill, what energy do I have to shop – shop?! – around and travel further than my local healthcare providers? What we want is to know that our local doctor, our local accident and emergency services, and our centres of speciality, will all of them offer good care. Do not give me, ignorant non-medic that I am, the choice of which cancer centre to go to. Who the blazes am I to judge whether Dr Matthew at Guy's is better than Dr Neil at UCLH? Train our healthcare professionals to an equal (within a reasonable spectrum) standard of professionalism and clinical wisdom. All of them, for heaven's sake. Surely that is the reasonable request? Or am I missing something?

Friday, 20 December

The journey to Hastings is gruelling. Flooding in Balcombe has tipped Southern railway passengers on to Southeastern, and though a landslip in Robertsbridge has been cleared enough to let our train slowly through I think we are the last because rail replacement buses populate Hastings Station forecourt when we finally disembark. Most of us, God bless us all, are cheerfully grumpy as the train crawls along, the poor guard telling us what he knows when he knows it, including how little he knows or is able to predict. Stuck at Etchingham Station for an extended period, he rather sweetly offers to keep an eye out if we want to disembark and have a smoke; he will make sure we don't get left behind. 'Thank you for choosing to travel with Southeastern.' Having a 'choice' about train operators makes no difference to the weather. The rain falls on all of us.

We are finally home. Making tea, I put sugar in my own cup instead of Seán's, and, quite suddenly, I fall apart. I weep, I can't breathe, I think I shall faint, I can't stand up. Shivering by the radiator in the kitchen, my tears fall for a long time. I'm not sure what is going on. Relief after the whole ordeal? Coming back to Hastings is a milestone in my recovery; perhaps I have unconsciously invested our arrival with a significance that, now it has been achieved, leaves me weak and helpless, all over again. Seán is characteristically wise: he lets me cry, rubs my back, says nothing, is not disturbed by the strange, strangled noises of my breathing and my weeping.

After supper we light a comforting fire. In *Silas Marner*, George Eliot advises Christianity to beware dismissing the fetishism of fire worship lest it cut off its own roots.

Saturday, 21 December

I sit up in bed writing this, in my Rupert Bear nightshirt, big yellow jumper, big yellow scarf, long yellow socks and a tawny corduroy beret on my exposed scalp, warm as toast under the duvet, looking at the view (I am touch-typing), as a wintry sun emerges from clouds, waves crash gloriously against the harbour arm, a few gulls cry in the valley of the Old Town. The sun's rays pierce the clouds and send shafts of benediction on to the sea; no softness here but a definite 'yes, I mean you' straight line of light; now the clouds cover it again but the sun is still there. The sun: another ancient source of worship Christianity would do well to respect. Worship. Or fear, if you are in Australia where fires rage. The sun shines on all, regardless. No choice there.

Sunday, 22 December

Yesterday was the shortest day. This morning I watch the late dawn, but it is a couple of minutes earlier than yesterday's. From now on, each day will be longer by about two minutes. It's a pleasing coincidence with my own gradual recovery.

The things that I must do to gain strength and stay alive and well – eat, sleep, wash, exercise, drink water, swallow pills – are imperceptibly receding into their quotidian place, and the things that give a life interest and flair and meaning are raising their tantalising heads: they have been in the interstices while the subsistence activities have taken centre stage. I think, though, that having to concentrate on the essentials, and having no energy for more than they, forces one to make of them something special: creativity in the food; care in the washing; interest in the exercise; attentive love in all of it. These quotidian roles are proper employment. Heaven knows we acknowledge (or should) the saintliness of those whose work is to keep the rest of us cared for and alive.

We go for a first glorious walk in the woods since my sojourn in hell. This is joy: back in nature, smelling the rich dampness of the fallen leaves, squelching in our gum boots through thick mud, clasping a tree trunk or each other for steadiness, breathing, walking, being.

Life wants to live. This is what I experienced at my lowest, death-like Melphalan ebb, feel in my own body now and also sense in nature, even as I pass through its wintry dying phase. Life wants to live. Not because humans will that it should; not because of something I do or want or say, but despite everything. Does this mean that the planet's ecological health will recover?

Thirty-second Letter

Dear Readers

I am pondering the fact that I've had to put my body first this year and put changing the world on the back burner; and how it would be good to work out how not to separate the two.

And I'm thinking about consent. I have argued in these letters that consent as legally defined is, for me, impossible. I am not (fully) competent, I am not adequately informed, and I am coerced into saying yes. Not by anyone else, but by the circumstances: if, like M the magician in the pork pie hat, I were to have galloping myeloma and were asked to have another stem cell transplant ten weeks after the first, even knowing what it entails now, God help me, I would still feel that I had to say yes. My agreement to the treatment is based more than anything else on my trust of the clinical team.

Now I think: This is true of all of my decisions. I make them based upon inadequate information, often feeling I have no choice, and often making them when less than clear in my own mind.

But consent still matters because I have to take moral responsibility for my acts, even though I'm only partly in control of them. I have to. It's like the difficulty of trying to live a life that doesn't harm the planet or other humans. I can only do so much with my purchasing choices and efforts to upcycle and recycle, turn down the heating, not fly, etc. Inevitably, I'm caught up in procurement chains and pension investment practices and all the other interwoven actions that make up a complex economy, actions that are at best morally blurred. But I still should feel morally responsible for my actions. It's no good shifting culpability elsewhere. We're caught up in the moral muddle together.

Tuesday, 24 December

I watch the dawn and wait for the sun but the sky is light and day has arrived long before the sun shows itself. Like God: I can't see God yet, but I am looking at God's works.

I feel sartorially bound to clarify that by 'Rupert Bear nightshirt' I did not mean that I was wearing a nightshirt covered in Rupert Bears. I was wearing a nightshirt in a fetching yellow tartan with black and red stripes. Nurse Anzie said it made her think of Rupert Bear.

The final reflection by Augustus in John Williams' eponymous novel[6] includes this thought: one is trying to make sense of the universe even as one is living through it. We will fail, but it's so interesting to try. That describes these diaries exactly. Thank you, G, for sending the book. It's brilliant, nearly as good as *Stoner*[7] but in a completely different way.

I climb back on a horse! A half-hour riding lesson. The school is outside and the Sussex hills are on glorious show in the wintry air. It is fabulous to be back on Nutkin again and feels just right. But I am weak physically and psychologically and not much good at getting her to trot and canter. Chloe, who is teaching us and is very kind, clicks and Nutkin responds to her.

In the High Street R says I have the shining look of one who is pregnant. C wants me to swim on new year's day (it's an Old Town custom) and when I tell him I'd better not on account of the vile chemotherapy he says I don't look as though I've had vile chemotherapy. I can't tell you how much these comments help.

Friday, 27 December

I wake up with a cold.

My body is pre-eminent. I thought convalescence, when you can't do too much, was a good opportunity to be spiritual, but in fact my body demands attention as it gets better and I can't settle to prayer with an unsettled body in the same way. I feel this is a failing but it is also a fact so I should at least learn from it. I can't meditate without a body, so I'd better attend to my body.

I revel in Tirzah Garwood's autobiography *Long Live Great Bardfield* (thank you, N).[8] She simply, effectively, evokes the detail of life in the 1920s to 1950s, married to Eric Ravilious, her part in his work, her own creativity and success, her acceptance of the pain of childbirth, the hard work of living through the war, and, later, the pain of cancer treatments. She is, as you say, N, such excellent company. Her writing is so delightfully unassuming and self-effacing (but not in a self-denigrating way) that she puts me to shame. It's been me, me, me all year. Even reading her by reference to my own writing is self-obsessed.

Saturday, 28 December

We are planning new year's eve. Because we have to go to bed early, we work out where in the world it would be midnight at 8.00pm our time, and choose Kazakhstan. We got the idea from neighbours who have a Mongolian new year (10.30pm); and I am now imagining, all around Hastings Old Town, people having different nationalities' new years depending on what time they want to go to bed. In preparation we play the Kazakh national anthem and practise what we imagine might be their army's high-stepping parading, saluting, eyes right, on the spurious grounds that lots of countries seem to have this. We don't last very long but neither does the national anthem. Our further research indicates that we need to wear turbans and eat, as well as furiously ride horses.

Sunday, 29 December

There has been a tragedy in Kazakhstan with a plane coming down. We will incorporate two minutes' silence into our evening.

Julian says she saw, contrary to the teaching of 'holy church', no damned souls, nor any sin, nor any wrath in God: if God were wrath even for one moment the whole of creation, held and kept by his love, would fail. That was the meaning of her famous hazelnut vision: all that is created, no greater than the size of a hazelnut lying in her palm, is kept, and ever shall be, by God's love.

It occurs to me that Tirzah Garwood is rather like Julian in her clear seeing and writing of what she experiences. Like Julian she will not deny what she sees, even if it flies in the face of convention, which might have felt equivalent to church teaching in her day.

Seán and I each name five blessings over our late breakfast egg. He tops my list and I, to my amazement, top his. Then I am struck by the way that a number of my blessings could be counted as curses. For example, not having any children. That could be felt as a curse. But it is also a blessing: with no dependants we are free to go wherever we are called.

Thirty-third Letter

Dear Readers

Our Kazakh new year's eve is tremendous. I find a purple corduroy full-length gown with buttons down the front, put bright yellow tights and tunic on underneath it and leave the buttons undone from the mid-thigh, add my faux fox-fur-Anna-Karenina hat and a necklace of gold coins, and tie a yellow sash round my waist. I think I look very well. I go into the kitchen and nearly die of fright to see, crouching down by the wine rack, a huge shaggy animal, sheep or something, in place of Seán's head. He stands up. He is wearing a hat about a foot-and-a-half across made of some steppe-creature's wool, and a Kazakh stiff-quilted long coat. It turns out that one of our neighbours, whom Seán bumped into earlier today, has visited Uzbekistan and Kazakhstan and had brought home these souvenirs. Though how he carried the hat through security I cannot imagine. I swear it is the size of a small sheep that hasn't been sheared, ever.

We watch *Borat*, Sacha Baron Cohen's film about Kazakhstan. It is in the category of cringe humour, like *Little Britain* or *The Office*, and Sacha Baron Cohen pushes the cringe beyond bearing until you give up and have to laugh as much at your own discomfort as at the utterly tasteless conversation or act that is being displayed on the screen. It is a very clever film indeed, revealing without rancour and with devastating honesty the appalling prejudices we will betray if the person we are speaking to makes us think he shares them.

We eat horsemeat stew. *Not!*

Wednesday, 1 January

An email sits in my inbox from Sarah, the clinical trial coordinator at Guy's with the first set of dates for my maintenance chemotherapy. I start again on 27 February. Eighteen months of chemotherapy. This coming year and beyond will be an endurance test: I look towards it and see a dreary need for patience. Will you stay the course with me, Dear Readers? I don't want to make more of it than it is, I'm really hoping it won't be painful or difficult, just tedious, but it's still another set of invasions into my poor body and it is going to go on for a long time. I hate the thought of it and I would welcome your companionship. Having that, I will be encouraged to make something of it that is at least a bit interesting, or funny even.

I ask Sarah if I can now have a port inserted, so that at least I won't have the weekly pain of cannulation. She checks, and tells me I can.

A second cranio-sacral session with Samvida in two days is deeply settling. She says my body is strong. We talk about letting things unfold in our lives. I have eighteen months ahead of me to practise patience and I feel a trust growing that all will be well, without knowing what that means.

Thursday, 2 January

In the disturbed night, tossing and turning as usual, a sense dawns that everything that is happening – my sweating, coughing body, the snuggly bedclothes, the still air, the deep night-time silence – are all God's love expressing itself, all the time, and there is nothing to worry about, nothing to achieve or deserve or discover.

The day dawns and light is everywhere though the sun itself has not appeared over the horizon. Now the sky and sea are half a dozen shades of grey, and the reddish-brown colours of the Old Town rooftops emerge in the strengthening light. A work-lorry blinks yellow flashes as it makes its winding way up past All Saints Street towards Tackleway on the East Hill. The gulls cry.

A clue in *The Oldie* Moron's Crossword: 'For good (11)'. I spend a long time trying to think of synonyms of 'forever'; but the answer is 'benignantly'. The conflating of 'forever' with 'good' pleases me.

We walk through the mud of Guestling Woods, our strong pace set by N, a pint of Guinness with a dish of whitebait at the pub two-thirds of the way along. Delicious.

I am training up for my next, endless chemotherapy round. I need to be physically strong and psychologically prepared, as anyone would need to be before a bodily challenge. Astronauts exposed to radiation do it: so should we cancer patients, if we can. Walking, riding, cranio-sacral therapy, acupuncture, Pilates, cycling when I'm back in London, swimming when it's warm enough. Meditation. They matter, Seán points out; they're not luxuries. There is more and more literature about so-called 'prehab' for chemotherapy and that is what I am about now, as my strength restores itself, emerging battered and bruised from the trauma of the transplant.

I go to Samvida and Weidong for cranio-sacral and acupuncture respectively, expecting to find the actual experience of the therapy enjoyable, relaxing and immediately restorative, as well as helping me in the long term. I go to chemotherapy expecting the horrid pain of cannulation in my wretched used and abused veins and receipt of a nasty substance that will make me feel sick, alleviated by the powerful kindness of the nurses. But the chemotherapy is given primacy by the fact of being life-saving in a way that complementary therapy is not and does not claim to be.

Friday, 3 January

Today is two weeks since I saw nurse Zoe; now, she said, my hair would start growing, and I peer at my still-visible scalp to see evidence of new shoots. My old hair is growing nicely, a silvery grey that I rather like and think I may cultivate, in consultation with my excellent hairdresser Judith, of course. But there isn't enough of it and more is needed. So come on, follicles, you heard what Zoe said.

I ride on lovely mare L'Arcelle, the sinuous movement of whose long back has my own hips swinging from side to side in response. You don't just sit on a horse when she walks ('like a sack of potatoes', Rachel observed of my riding when I first started with her), you actively move with her. L'Arcelle makes me feel like a model on the catwalk.

Sunday, 5 January

I am wrapped in the warmth and goodwill particularly of the women of Hastings at your party, N, in an atmosphere you create with your own generosity and kind heart. I take courage, and remove my beret, and receive the inevitable glances softly because they come with love as well as curiosity.

Later at home I keep touching my head, thinking I am wearing a hat, but I'm not. I can feel something. Are my follicles up and at it??

Thirty-fourth Letter

Dear Readers

Monday, 6 January

I try to buy a book online, deeply irritated by how my attention is pestered by algorithmic suggestions of other goods based upon previous online searches, the website's default settings to include me in subscription deals, the website's default storing of my credit card details, and more. It feels like walking through a market in Egypt: I once had to buy a scarf against the sun there but had little time to spare, so I chose the scarf I wanted from a distance, before the sellers had noticed me, went straight to it and asked to buy it, offered a price about a third below what was asked, and responded *la, shukram* (no, thank you) with a big smile to the ubiquitous, numerous, importunate attempts to sell me more scarves and other good things both in the stall and as I made my way back to the bus. The moment your interest is piqued, and your attention turns to something other than the thing you want to buy, you are lost. My determination earned the admiration of the bus driver.

I need focused attention for study, and I need wide attention for swimming and riding. They are a priceless gift because they give me energy, they don't deprive me of it. Attention pulled in many directions, with no strength in me to keep it from darting about in response, is exhausting.

Dreaming and distraction are really important too, but maybe not online.

The Dear Readers' playlist is such a joy because as well as introducing me to music of which I have never heard and music of which

205

I have heard but never listened to, as each piece plays it brings you who chose it to mind, enriching the experience. Not 'What this algorithm has worked out you will like, Claire', but 'What I, who care about you, love myself'. Relationship quickened to life, not exhaustion from pestered attention.

Wednesday, 8 January

In London, enjoying its anonymity and activity as I move more slowly, noticing more.

Friday, 10 January

The rippling joy of a ride on L'Arcelle. I test my strength: today I can stand up in my saddle trotting up the lane which is a good indication of a functioning abdominal transverse muscle corset.

Sunday, 12 January

Am I beautiful? I weep in Seán's arms. Shorn of hair, androgynous, I don't feel like a sexual being.

And my confidence in writing to you, Dear Readers, drains away. Why should I subject you to my endless wittering? Surely you've done enough reading service in the last year and it's time for me to keep my thoughts to myself? I send no letter, and go to bed depressed.

Monday, 13 January

I think of the steady professionalism of my writer friends like Laura Wilson who unfussily turns up for work and delivers, and pull myself together. I will keep writing. I'm sad when I don't, and you are kind. I send this letter.

And I also think that the message my laptop keeps blinking at me: 'Your startup disk is almost full' could be delivered to my own psyche. I have been reborn, because of the stem cell transplant, but with a head full of notions already of what my life is to be.

A Pilates session reminds me to listen to my body, not talk to it.

Thirty-fifth Letter

Dear Readers

Tuesday, 14 January

This is the cost of too-focused attention. Waiting on the platform at Hastings for the train doors to unlock (it is a terminus so the train stands for some time), I become engrossed in writing an email, do not notice when the doors unlock, and only come to when the guard blows his whistle. I am too late, frantically pressing the 'open' button on the door. The guard is implacable and the train leaves without me. And I had arrived ten minutes before it was due to depart. I tell the guard he is cruel but it is more than his job is worth to let the train leave late, even seconds late, he says. It is not the guard who is cruel.

Wednesday, 15 January

To the Saatchi Gallery to meet Seán and see the Tutankhamun exhibition. I cycle from Borough on the south side of the river to Chelsea Bridge through the building site of the US embassy in Nine Elms. The embassy has a high, impervious wall around it, like other walls we could mention. Mr Trump spurned the invitation to open the building, saying it should not have moved from prime real estate territory in Belgravia to so low class a part of London, but the embassy has brought its own cachet with it so Nine Elms is now, or is going to be, very smart indeed. It doesn't feel in the least bit welcoming; it is not human-sized. Everything rears up grandly and turns blind square sides to the road; everything is private, hermetically sealed. I just checked that I had the right word 'cachet' and am delighted by the discovery that not only does it mean prestigious, it also means a flat capsule containing a dose of unpleasant medicine. I think that is an excellent description of what Nine Elms is becoming. A snippet from a Radio 4 programme is relevant: 'Our world is becoming too smooth'.

I harbour a great fondness for the area because Seán and I had a first sort-of date here, at a jazz concert on the Battersea Barge when it was much less smart.

There are cycle lanes around Vauxhall Bridge on the south side, and on and off all along my route to and across Chelsea Bridge, but they are, infuriatingly, both insistent (you have to use them; there is no spare room where the cars are) and also deeply confusing.

Later, after choir and the pub, with not a Sadiq cycle to hire in sight, I walk back to the flat, past the Museum of London to St Paul's, watching a fox who lingers on the pavement, looking around. The dome of the Cathedral glows above him as he slowly trots over to some bin bags, sniffs and pees, just like a dog. He crosses the road and sniffs at more bin bags. He is at home here, slender, elegant with his bushy tail and pointed nose. Unafraid. I walk on, left into Cheapside, down Bow Lane to Southwark Bridge. I feel like the fox, at home.

Friday, 17 January

This morning, quite suddenly, my eyebrows are sprouting. They grow in abundance where my tattooed eyebrows are not, so a prolonged and painful period of tweezer-plucking ensues. The hairs are immediately quite long – how does that happen? No such sprouting on my scalp, that I can see, but it is definitely more grey, less pink. Shall I have iron grey hair?

The ride! I am on Denby again, and he, like the other horses, is full of energy. As we turn into the dell where the horses know they are up for a run, Denby pulls ahead, charging in front of the other horses. Sophie, just behind on Wooster, eggs us on: 'Head up, Claire, heels down, shoulders back, now go! You wanted a run, Denby, go for it!' And Denby goes: this is an actual gallop. I love Sophie for trusting me and relax because of it, loving the speed and power . . . Then Denby does a sort of sideways leap which really nearly throws me. Spattered with mud from the pony Sky who had been in front for an earlier canter, now Denby spatters those who ride behind as his hoofs fly over the wet ground. We race on until the track runs out near the top of the field; Sophie now in front, bringing the whole group down to a trot and then a walk, and quietly turning us all into the wind and towards home. It turns out that Denby's leap was an attempt to kick Wooster to stop him overtaking, a high kick at his flank. No wonder I nearly came off. Equally exciting things had been happening further back in the group, and everyone is exhilarated, delighted to have been in on the powerful gallop, letting the horses have their head, giving them the chance to expel their pent-up winter energy. Going with the flow. Sophie says that if you can stay on, and she was confident this group of riders would, and the way is clear, it is much safer to let the horses go than to try and control them, powerful beasts that they are, so much stronger than we. She also tells me that Rachel had instructed her to make sure I have a quiet ride because I'm not well. But this poor cancer victim, trying to find the equanimity to face the next long, long round of treatment, has been startled into the sheer joy of letting nature take her course. I am completely alive and laughing, heart thumping, on my mettle, engaged and free, and Sophie, confident enough to let me face the potential danger, can see this.

Later, after a hot bath has washed away the mud, I stand at the window high up in the house and look at the sea and the waves sparkling as they crash against the harbour arm again and again, and I think of King Cnut demonstrating his inability to control the water; and I wonder why I fret about things.

Sunday, 19 January

I have only just learned this week that 'bucket list' is called that because of the phrase 'kicking the bucket', hence what you want to do before you die.

I reread the list I wrote at the time of my diagnosis, and I think: how modest.

Now, after a year of having to put my body first, putting nature first, matter over mind rather than mind over matter, and finding joy in the reversion, I would add this to the list: to find a way for the human family to live on this planet without harming it.

I want to defy the defeatism that thinks we have to choose between serving ourselves and serving nature. If we think that way, it will be the human family that loses out, not nature.

The task requires creative endeavour on so many levels.

For me, I think the work is to use words to awaken our perception of the divinity in our world. The enchanting beauty of existence that both is love and kindles love, which in turn kindles the desire to serve. I see it, Dear Readers! It shines. It shines.

Thirty-sixth Letter

Dear Readers

Monday, 20 January

Waiting on the platform at London Bridge I am delighted to see a woman wearing a houndstooth patterned face mask and immediately want one.

Tuesday, 21 January

It is a quiet ride in clear bright air softened by sunshine. I am on Wooster who is calm today – all the horses are. Mostly we are in deeply restful silence, which gives me time and space to receive the world we move through.

Wednesday, 22 January

I am having such a brilliant time with colour. I start by choosing the hat I am going to wear (I have rather a lot now, thanks mainly to the Hat Shop in Hastings Old Town). Today: the mustard yellow cap. Then I select the rest of my outfit, with as bright colours as possible in my lovely autumn palette. Mustard yellow baggy trousers; chestnut brown top, big mustard yellow scarf. I did one of those colour consultations a few years ago and I cannot tell you how valuable an investment it has turned out to be. I carefully apply make up. Hairlessness obliges me to make an effort. And I really want to stay a few pounds lighter: this could be Melphalan's lasting, welcome gift to me. Just a few pounds lighter makes an enormous difference, out of all proportion to what it physically is. I love it.

I am also having a brilliant time with George Orwell: it's the seventieth anniversary of *1984*'s publication and there's a lot about him on the radio. I am writing about truth-telling in public life so I reread his essay 'Politics and the English Language'. I agree with his argument for clarity of language, and share his suspicion of unclear language. Laziness in language can lead to corruption in politics as obfuscation creeps in and more sinister intentions are hidden by unchallenged propaganda. Dead phrases and over-used metaphors anaesthetise part of the brain. When I am editing my own work I ask, over and over again: Is this really what I mean? And when I am writing *de novo* I ask the question: What am I really trying to say?'

But no, George, I am not going to jettison words that are not Anglo-Saxon, like *de novo*: it's too beautiful and mellifluous. And I am going to use long ones. Words like mellifluous and obfuscate are glorious and I want to use them. I am Parrot in Gerald Durrell's *Talking Parcel*: I believe that words need outings and they come to life if well placed. Not to show off (well not much), and certainly not to obfuscate (there you are). But the English language is rich in synonyms and words from other languages; it is strong and prolific and mongrel, and all the better for it. It's a bit like adorning one's body well: not to hide it but to glorify it.

Names of things matter. When does mass murder become genocide? When does a refugee become an asylum seeker? When does treatment become torture? (When it's Melphalan or a bone marrow biopsy.)

We go to the Lucien Freud exhibition of his self-portraits. I am struck by his phrase 'biological truth-telling'. He was such an honest depicter of the human form, and here we see him developing his style, using himself as a practice model; being, then, pitilessly honest about himself before he was then pitiless with his other models. But Pope Benedict's sentiment applies, I think: truth is vital but without love it is unbearable. Freud is not kind.

Friday, 24 January

I ride L'Arcelle. She is grumpy. The air is muffled by low cloud that seems portentous. We have a good run, one of the fields is not too muddy so there is plenty of cantering, but we finish in the riding school for an extra canter, and, in my case, humiliation. In the school one's true horsewomanship is exposed, because we take it in turns to walk, trot and canter and everyone else watches. On a hack the horses just do what the one in front does. In the school the rider is supposed to be in charge. Not me, not on L'Arcelle, who does not take my instruction: I barely raise a trot and only achieve a canter because Sophie is now standing nearby and L'Arcelle obeys her voice.

There is an amount of literature and public discussion of the value of going with the menstrual flow – using the different phases of the month's cycle to work most happily and efficiently. It reminds me of the scuba diving principle, following the same swimming pattern as the fish. When the tide sweeps you forward, you swim. When it washes back, you let it take you. You still make headway, still arrive at your destination, but you make progress with the flow of nature, not against it. So, then, I think, if menstrual cycles can be creative, what of the hot flushes of the menopause? What is the flow to be followed here? They are hot and uncomfortable, the physical discomfort always preceded, in my case, by emotional upset and irritation. The only good in them that I can discern is that they will pass. They themselves have no value at all, I feel, except probably a hidden one, rebalancing something in my body, at least they better had.

Today I think this: hot flushes teach me patience and compassion. I have to wait until the wave of anxiety then irritation passes; I am learning not to speak or act from their stabbing motivation. And to be kind to myself while I'm hot, moving slowly, as one does in a hot climate. It's the same as with the matter–over–mind experience of treatment: there are times when I am rendered powerless, and I have to wait until my power returns, patiently and with kindness. Rather than being outraged at my body's uncalled-for discomfort, I set my mind to learn from it.

★   ★   ★

I meet Seán off the London train. He has had a bronchoscopy this morning. He is tired, and I enjoy being the carer for a change.

Sunday, 26 January

I sit up in bed and undertake half an hour of meditation using *maranatha*. At last some time dedicated purely and simply to God. It is such a relief: I have missed it; but the new life activating in me seemed to preclude this kind of quiet and stillness. I have re-inserted it. I consciously summon my capacity for the kind of focus that makes me miss trains and, for a little while, I am dead to the world.

Thirty-seventh Letter

Dear Readers

The cancer-treatment-related faff recommences. I go to Guy's so Sarah can take blood and swabs before booking the operation for my port to be inserted. It's lovely to see her, but my heart quails as I am jolted back into the truth that I have cancer and I am not even half-way through my treatment.

You ask yourself, C, what you have been doing all your life, and your answer is: 'work'. That is my answer too. I have recently been forced by circumstance to recalibrate my life away from being work-centred, in order to make it health-centred, but now that I am gearing up to be back actively as Director of Westminster Abbey Institute, not just in-the-background Director, all my long-lived habits of thought return. I see my diary fill up again, engagements jostling, appointments lined up, no space between them, and everything to do with my health — treatment, meditation, keeping fit — relegated to the interstices. And my anxiety rises like a spring tide.

This will not do. I have set my mind to be taught by my body's needs, to learn patience and compassion. But how, *how* do we who love our work, which is vocational and hence deeply defines us, which is creative and expansive like a person whom one loves more and more, work that makes us grow and think harder and respond afresh, how do we keep a balance? When I am weak, I have no choice but to step back. But now I grow strong again, so where and how do I set limits?

★   ★   ★

I remember walking along Tufton Street towards St James's Park station one day, when I was still medical and environmental ethics adviser to the Church of England, thinking about genetic engineering, and being stopped in my tracks by the verse from the Sermon on the Mount that entered my head like a bullet: 'Which of you by taking thought can add one cubit unto his stature?' (Matthew 6:27, KJV). I stood still as a stone on Tufton Street, deep in thought, the crowds flowing around and past me. I didn't hear the verse as an injunction against genetic engineering, I heard it as a statement of our physical limits. However much we try, genetically or otherwise, we cannot make ourselves able to be in more than one place at the same time. However many luxury homes we may be able to afford to build around the world, we cannot be in more than one of them at a time; we may have a dozen speedy cars but we cannot drive more than one at a time; we cannot sit in more than one private cinema at a time; exercise in more than one gym; fly in more than one private jet plane; and so on. Money will not overcome the limitations of our bodies.

Technology appears to be overcoming those limits. For example, you can watch a film and be involved in several online conversations in different corners of the same screen. But that way madness lies. Madness to try to live as though we have added cubits to our stature and can enjoy doing more than one thing at a time.

So, yes, I am limited by my physicality, and however much my mind can soar to the heights of possibilities for my work with the Institute, my body binds me to the Earth.

An ambitious king who wanted to save the world and achieve enlightenment consulted a wise old priest. 'What do I need to do to achieve my goals?' he asked. 'Sleep for as long as possible,' she replied, immediately. 'How can I serve others and develop spiritually if I am asleep?' asked the king. 'I don't know,' said the priest. 'But it will give the Earth and all of us a rest.'

> For there it lies so tranquil . . .
> So gentle, stirless, helpless, and unmoved . . .
> All it hath felt, inflicted, pass'd and proved,
> Hush'd into depth . . .[9]

Satish Kumar had the brilliant idea of 'fossil-free sabbaths'. On your sabbath day, whatever you engage in, let it not involve the use of fossil fuels. Walking, for example. Having a conversation. Digging the garden.

So I say to myself in response to my rising anxiety: Stop. Put your body first (which is, after all, a microcosm of putting the Earth first). Trust that what needs to be done will be done, not all of it by you. You will give your team and Westminster Abbey a rest . . .

Wednesday, 29 January

At my desk at the flat in Borough, I run out to say hello to the tots who walk past each day from their nursery to the park. I still have the card they made me on my desk, cheering me up. C, their head, tells me to keep smiling. The tots are delightful, perfect little diminutives, fatly waving from their tightly buttoned coats.

Later we go to the exhibition on light in Rembrandt's art at Dulwich Picture Gallery. I spend a long time in front of *Entombment*. This is a simple sketch of the dead Christ being laid into Joseph of Arimathea's tomb, in a dark cave, surrounded by people; the light falls upon Christ's face and Mary, bending over him. It is like a pietà.

Rembrandt paints his people thinking. This gives his art even more honesty than Freud's because even more of what and who the person is is depicted, not just the harsh reality of the physical condition but also the interior life. It's more revealing. And kind. I think Rembrandt loves his sitters. He doesn't objectify them, which Freud does. There's truth but it is bearable.

I would love to be painted by Rembrandt.

Thursday, 30 January

Seán's bronchoscopy has produced some results. He has haemophilus influenzae. It can be treated with antibiotics.

Your quotation, G, sheds light on the unfolding of these letters:

In following a story we follow a storyteller or more precisely, we
follow the trajectory of a storyteller's attention, what it notices

and what it ignores, what it lingers on, what it repeats, what it considers irrelevant, what it hurries towards, what it circles, what it brings together . . . we become accustomed to the storyteller's particular procedure of bestowing attention and then of making a certain sense of what at first glance was chaotic.[10]

I don't have much confidence in what I write, I just love to do it; it helps me inordinately and I am so grateful that you receive it. I struggle, and inevitably fail, to make as much sense as I would like to, but my search for meaning has resulted in all these words. At the exhibition of Gaugin's portraits at the National Gallery, I found myself really grateful to have the chance to see what he regarded as the detritus of his failed search for purity, detritus that is, in fact, powerful and extraordinary work. We leave each other the by-product of our failed searches, so thank heavens we embark on these searches!

One hundred days since my transplant. I have my exit interview with Dr Neil at UCLH. I cycle there, because I can, but also so that I can boast of the evidence of my restored energy. As I tell him, the doctors hear the best of us, we do all we can to put on a good face for them, wanting praise and recognition for our wellness, as if overcoming symptoms was a competition. So they don't really hear the truth from us. I offer to send him my account of the stem cell transplant, and he agrees. He is a truly humane doctor.

Friday, 31 January

I have a lesson with Sophie instead of a ride and I learn a lot. We practise walking with the horse, letting his rolling gait lead ours so our left buttock moves when his does, our right when his does, our lower back softened by the movement. If we want to stop, we have to stop moving our bottoms and squeeze them, before doing anything else like pulling the reins or saying whoa. Even Denby, my horse for the lesson, begins to slow down at this very subtle act of physical direction. We practise this from trotting too. And we learn different seats in cantering; one raised and forward, the other seated and upright, again moving with the horse, not bumping up and down as he leaps forward. Sophie bellows encouragement when I feel I'm getting nowhere, and shouts in delight when I find my seat and Denby and I move as one, for a very little while. It is quite magical when that happens. So much flows from relaxing and moving with the horse, doing as little as possible, being as stable as possible. We are tuning in to each other, Sophie says. More great metaphors for humans and our interaction with the environment.

Having gone to bed early, I awaken at 11.00pm, as a few desultory fireworks go off on the Fishermen's Beach. We're out of the EU. So much speculation about what would happen, so much to discover, now, of what actually happens. Isn't it gorgeously ironic that we left at 11.00pm, which is European midnight, not our midnight?

Saturday, 1 February

I have a proper fuzzy covering of hair on my head. It's so exciting. I keep brushing it with the flat of my hand. For information, if I meet any of you, I am really pleased to have my head brushed like that, having always found it difficult to resist the temptation to do it to other heads of similar hair. So do go ahead (ha). Also, since it only takes about a nanosecond to get used to what I look like now, offering my head to be stroked gives you the time you need to adjust. My bent, proffered head and downcast eyes mean you don't have to try and make your faces behave for that initial moment of shock, because I'm not looking at you, so you can let your face look what you feel. And I am protected from seeing pity in your eyes, which I don't really like. Well, I do sometimes.

Sunday, 2 February

I finish *Barnaby Rudge*. A closing speech by Mr Haredale, a Catholic whose property is destroyed by the Gordon rioters, strikes me as good advice in the contrary:

I have had my share of sorrows — more than the common lot, perhaps, but I have borne them ill. I have broken where I should have bent; and have mused and brooded, when my spirit should have mixed with all God's great creation. The men who learn endurance are they who call the whole world brother. I have turned from the world, and I pay the penalty.[11]

I haven't had my property mindlessly destroyed but I am facing more physical invasions, and I really hope I can carry on bending and brothering and mixing with all God's creation, in this next period.

Thirty-eighth Letter

Dear Readers

Monday, 3 February

I ponder the liberating and slightly nerve-racking experience of meeting any of you, Dear Readers, face to face now that I have been writing to you for so long. I have shown you my most honest and innermost thoughts, feelings and experiences, so I cannot pretend to be other than who I am when I see you.

A delicious new word found in Omand's *Securing the State*:[12] a '*schlimazel*', someone to whom the worst always happens.

We are going to Rome for a few days before chemotherapy begins again. I pack, but it doesn't take very long, as we are too mean to buy more allowance than one piece of hand luggage. What can I not do without? I find this question, and the resulting handbag-sized luggage, very pleasing and relieving. We will travel light. Of course, it helps a great deal that I don't have to pack any hair effects: hair dryer, mousse, brushes. Just a tiny bottle of shampoo to share with Seán.

Tuesday, 4 February

We are on the 4.00am night bus to Liverpool Street station. The bus is packed. Packed. Sleepy workers; where there is talk it is all not-English. These are the cleaners and coffee-makers and porters keeping the City financiers going. It beggars belief, the contrast between the lives of these people and the places they flow into each morning at this early hour. We are NOT different species but by heavens we behave as if we are.

In Rome

Seán is deeply unhappy about the design of our modest room in a tall building behind the Piazza Navona. Especially the bathroom. The sink is too large; the lavatory too near; the edges of everything, including the door handles, too sharp. Clearly a lot of thought has gone into the design; it is meant to be modern and clean. But it doesn't work; it is not comfortable; the lights are all in the wrong place; and Seán is unhappy in the way a teacher would be unhappy seeing the potential in a child going to waste.

We spend a day at the Vatican. Going into the basilica of St Peter, we pay our respects to Michelangelo's pietà, which moves me deeply. Walking into the huge space of the church, my spirit expands, receiving it. We visit the tomb of St Peter, and I have the same response as I had at the holy sites in Israel–Palestine. Sudden depth, tears, touching eternity for a quick moment; a gift from all the millions who have come before and offered their devotion.

In the entrance to the crypt where Peter and so many of the popes are buried, there is a panel on which are carved all the names of the popes, ending with John Paul II and beginning with . . . St Peter. An extraordinary claim; attestation to and 'proof' of apostolic succession.

The Vatican museums are vast and full and wonderful. I am impressed and disturbed by the abiding sense of the triumphant claim of the Church to have embraced everything: the past in ancient civilisations; the future in scientific experimentation; the heavens; the deeps; all nations; all cultures.

An Etruscan perfume jar of a panther clasping her babe is like the Madonna, five centuries earlier.

A long corridor of sarcophagi from classical times, and then Christian ones mimicking the style but with Christian themes. You can tell which story is being depicted if you know which figure is Jesus: with jars (Cana); with a woman touching the hem of his robe (woman with issue of blood); with a young girl rising from a bed (Jairus' daughter); with a man with a bed on his back ('take up your bed and walk'); with a little man in a tree (Zaccheus); and so on.

A moving small statue of Christ the good shepherd, a very early depiction: clean shaven, standing like David, young, physically beautiful.

It is a long walk to the Sistine Chapel, passing through room after room of treasures. We take our time with Raphael; famous paintings seen in the flesh here, especially, for me, the painting of Philosophy with Plato in conversation with Aristotle, Socrates looking froglike, Euclid drawing geometry on a slate, Pythagoras teaching a group of disciples. There is a remarkable collection of modern art, including Bacon, our very own (Hastings') Sutherland, and a crucifix which I particularly love, utterly spare, just three pieces of wood, but the shape suggests Christ embracing the world.

We spend a long time in the Sistine Chapel, enjoying deciphering the characters and the stories in the paintings, and falling into conversation with a beautiful Muslim woman who wants to hear the stories too. She tells us that she named her son Isaac and gets into trouble for this, since it was not Isaac but his half brother Ishmael who is the founding prophet of Islam.

We spend a day in the Jewish quarter. Cities have layers of histories, none more so than Rome, and the Jewish story is compelling. There have been Jews in Rome since 200 BC; more sent there from Jerusalem when Titus destroyed the Temple in AD 70; more again, mainly Spanish, in 1492 with the edict of Ferdinand and Isabella banishing Jews from all their dominions; more again in 1967, mainly Libyan, after the Six-Day War. (There are now no Jews in Libya, whose culture there was ancient, thriving and distinctive.) Rome is the only city from which Jews have never been banished. But there was discrimination and persecution and between 1550 and 1870 the Jews were confined to a ghetto measuring 250 by 200 metres, alongside the Tiber river next to Marcello's theatre, where we are now. The land sat below the level of the water so every winter the ghetto flooded. Only one synagogue was permitted so five were hidden within one building. Jews were allowed to do no work except to lend money and deal in second-hand clothing. One pope banned memorial stones for the Jewish dead, so instead mantles for the sacred Torah scrolls, sewn together and exquisitely embroidered by women from the leftover rags of their trade, were donated in the name of their family members who had died, each carefully recorded, so even today a family can trace its ancestors back two or three hundred years through the carefully preserved historic Torah mantles. That pope failed to obliterate their names and memories, on the contrary. Italian unification in 1870 meant the pope no longer had secular rulership over Rome and the Jews were again free to live anywhere, to work, and to build synagogues. The Great Synagogue which we are visiting was built in 1904 and retains two of the altars from the old five-synagogue building, as a reminder.

In 1938 racial laws were drawn up, first against the colonial immigrants from Abyssinia, then against the Jews. Then with Nazi occupation in 1943 a deal was struck. The story is heartbreaking. If the Jewish community could produce fifty kilograms of gold within forty-eight hours, there would be no deportations to the camps. Every Jew in Rome brought what they had, from rings to cups to coins. The weight of gold was produced; the deportations happened anyway. There were 10,000 Jews in Rome at the time; 8,000 were hidden in convents and elsewhere; 2,000 were sent to the camps. The occupation only lasted until the following year so it was possible to keep the Jews hidden for that time. Many Christians helped to hide the Jews though Pope Pius XII famously failed to condemn the Holocaust. In 2021 the Vatican Archives will open to reveal what part, if any, he played behind the scenes; the Chief Rabbi Zolli converted to Catholicism after the war, and took Pius' birth name, Eugenius, in honour of him, but was it only Zolli whom Pius helped? We ask Ursula, our guide, about these things, and learn how very controversial the stories still are.

I sit under the dome of the Great Synagogue and look up at the rainbow depicted there; signifying G-d's promise to humankind. It feels the same blessing as the Holy Spirit in St Agnes in the Piazza Navona, to me.

I am not Jewish in Ursula's eyes, and I feel her rejection. I have felt this before, visiting the Jewish quarter in Prague; the same in

Amsterdam; less so in Venice and Ortigia but we didn't talk to anyone there. Your mother was not Jewish and you are not a Jew, Claire. But my Jewish blood sings so loudly: I cannot deny it even if other Jews do. Is my family history of persecution and flight immaterial? I feel the tragedy and experience the grief but I can only nurse it in my own heart, I cannot share it: there is no fellow feeling and I find this extremely painful. You are wholly one of us or you are not, and you, Claire, are not.

In honour of my ancestors and my living Jewish family, we dine at the most Jewish restaurant in the quarter we can find, eating unutterably delicious fried artichoke, salt cod in rich, heavy tomato sauce, fried endive, roast potatoes, and we drink Barkan red wine from the Holy Land.

If truth be told, I don't want to belong to any exclusive club. I hate being excluded from anywhere, but if the price of membership and welcome is to exclude others, I don't really want to join. Lovely Catholic church in Hastings, then, lovely Fr Eamonn, for letting me come in and showering such powerful blessings on my poor shaven head, without asking me to join properly. Lovely Church of England for its porosity.

And most of us, whoever we are, mourn deeply the horrific treatment that humanity has afflicted on others in the Holocaust and throughout our history; share the grief; acknowledge the tragedy. In our long history, no one is just a victim, none just a perpetrator.

Saturday, 8 February

Back from Rome, we go to hear exquisite Caccini's *Eurydice*, and Carissimi's *Jonah and Jephthah*, the earliest operas, first performed in 1610 and 1650 respectively. Sung by horribly beautiful and talented young singers in the echoing neo-Gothic Christ Church, St Leonard's, which makes me think of the Pitti Palace where *Eurydice* was first performed. The performance and the music are so spare. We love it.

A, who is sitting with us, strokes my head, and kisses it. 'It feels like a fruit,' she says in her still-strong Italian accent.

Sunday, 9 February

The wind soughs round the house, the waves batter the harbour arm. The alarm sounds warning that the lifeboat is to launch. We can hear it all the way back here on the West Hill. Lord, that will be a rough sea for the lifeboat people; and who or what are they saving?

V

Maintenance Chemotherapy and Covid-19

Thirty-ninth Letter

Dear Readers

It takes time to cultivate habits: could I use the next eighteen months to seriously cultivate the good life? Not by imposing more oughts in my life, but by releasing myself from many oughts. Learning to tune in, let go, breathe, smile and dance. Why not have a go? It will make something positive from my protracted treatment. The treatment goes on for too long just to be something I have to endure and get through, putting myself on hold until it is finished. Eighteen months. Today that feels impossible to see beyond.

But in flagrant contravention of my new resolve to learn from my body and move at the pace of nature, I have agreed to a week of painful operations. Today a bone marrow biopsy; on Wednesday my port will be inserted; on Thursday I am to have another PET/CT scan; and on Friday my maintenance chemotherapy infusions begin. How did I end up with so many invasive procedures stacked up back to back? I agreed to them. I thought it would be good to get them over with and get started on the chemotherapy. Why? In order to finish as soon as I could? Then what?

We stagger back on the train to London from Hastings, dodging trees that have fallen on the line and looking askance at passengers who sneeze possibly coronavirus at us, in time for a little lunch, but I feel rather sick.

My biopsy is at 2.00pm. There will be a long delay. One of the two rooms used for biopsies is taken out of action as it is needed to isolate a patient who is unwell, raising eyebrows and blood pressures: is it Covid-19?

I am finally called at around 4.15pm by a young woman who looks as though she is on her gap year. My heart quails. You do not want your biopsies undertaken by beginners. I can't help asking her how much experience she's had. Oh Lord, she only started last week, but she tells me brightly that she has done lots of other procedures, like tracheotomies, and is 'rated well' (saints preserve us from this language; am I to ask her what her score out of five is??). She is confident (the youngest doctors often are) and not thrown by my questioning. Her registrar will be with her, observing, she says, and will take over if necessary (if things go wrong??). 'Two for the price of one,' the registrar says when she appears. She looks only very slightly older, as though she might just have graduated.

Gas and air are not apparent, but the canister is produced when I ask for them, trying not to panic. I ask the doctors if they are aware how strong my cortex is, making the procedure particularly tough, but they look blank. That was supposed to have been in my notes.

On to the bed, into a foetal position, so the doctor can get at my lower back. I am clutching the gas and air handle and taking deep breaths through the plastic mouthpiece. I swallowed some co-codamol earlier (some of you need to close your eyes to read this) and some paracetamol, but it was so long ago that I doubt any analgesic effects linger.

The younger doctor confidently identifies where she is to 'go in'. The first part of the procedure, in which aspirate or proto-blood samples are withdrawn, is utterly horrible but not as utterly horrible as it has been in the past. I tell her so.

Then she goes 'back in' to collect some of the trefoil, the honeycomb structure of the bone marrow. This takes a long time and is FUCKING AGONY. Everything in me is curled up in tight, self-protecting tension: my body, my feet, my hands, one grasping the pillow, the other the gas and air handle, and I am biting on the mouthpiece so hard I fear my teeth will break.

'AAARGH. AAAARGH!' I shout. 'Do you want me to stop?' asks the younger doctor. 'NO!' I say. 'I'll make a noise but don't stop.' I'm quieter now, I want to encourage her — for crying out loud, why am I worrying about the doctor's state of mind? But it helps me. 'Please don't stop.'

On we go. 'AAAARGH. AAAAARGH!' This is so awful. I weep mascara on to the pillow as every cell in my body winces away from the pain. 'AAAARGH!' 'Don't worry,' says the registrar. What? I'm not shouting because I'm worried. I'm shouting because it HURTS LIKE CRAZY.

A pause. The doctors are whispering to each other. 'It's clot,' says one. 'CLOT??' I say, overhearing. Clot means blood not bone marrow sample. The registrar says, 'We have two options, Claire.' I let her go no further. 'I'm not coming back,' I say. 'Please finish the task.'

More local anaesthetic. And in goes the registrar, making a new, agonising hole. I am giddy with sucking at the gas and air and in my own private hell, not replying to questions about how I am. I'll look after myself, I think, you concentrate on what you have to do. But then the registrar asks me who my consultant is and I wonder if she is concerned that I'm going under, so I reply, slurring, 'Genghis Khan' (not really). I am conscious but I don't want to engage with the real world because my real world, at this moment, is unbearable.

The sample – a nice long worm of bone marrow structure – is finally retrieved. I try and say something about feeling connected to the sisterhood who suffer pain in childbirth, but I don't think the doctors have a clue what I'm on about. I don't think I do either. They tell me that I am more sensitive than most, who don't feel anything once the needle penetrates the bone beyond the cortex, while I am still roaring with pain, but what do they know? Lots of people have bone pain, like both my parents. I weep afresh for them. I am a wreck.

I am left to recover. A nurse will come and check my blood pressure and make sure I am all right to go home. I am cold so I climb under the blanket I have been lying on. I lie there for ages. I need the lavatory. Surely someone should be in by now. It is 5.45pm.

Finally, I get up and find the loo, seeing Seán who sits in lonely isolation in the deserted waiting room. I wave at him as I pass. I had better find a nurse to check me out before we leave. There are abject apologies. It seems everything is a bit up the creek this afternoon. I am angry but it is no one's fault — no one's fault I have to have a bone marrow biopsy, no one's fault it was so bloody awful, no one's fault that doctors have to be trained, no one's fault that messages didn't get through and I might have been left all night . . .

I have this biopsy because the Cardamon trial wants clear before and after measurements, not because I need it. If those who designed the trial had ANY IDEA how awful the bone marrow biopsy is surely they wouldn't demand them. But pain is only suffered by the patient. It is completely personal. The doctors in the room try to be kind but they cannot know the pain, only I can. Pay attention, medical profession, as you dole out Melphalan because 'it works', or design research protocols with multiple bone marrow biopsies because these give you neater measurements than blood or pee. You do not bear the cost, only reap the benefits.

Tuesday, 11 February

N, thank you for the etymology of *schlimazel:* a typical Yiddish combination of Hebrew *mazel* meaning 'luck' (as in *mazeltov*) and German *schlim* meaning 'slim'. And S and L, for the joke: a *schlemiel* is one who always spills the soup, while a *schlimazel* is the one it always lands on.

And thank you, W, for reminding me that once something has taken place, like my bone marrow biopsy, it is just a thought. Today I am sore, but the agony is firmly in the past.

We are saying 'Take care!' to each other as we take our leave these days, like a little spell or prayer against the coronavirus.

Wednesday, 12 February

Today the port is to be inserted in my chest. It is to be done under local anaesthetic but because I may need sedation for the pain I have to fast, no food or drink including water, for six hours before the operation.

I set the alarm and rise at 3.30am for a bowl of granola and a cup of tea. At 9.00am we settle in the uncomfortable waiting area in the interventional radiology department at Guy's, with music playing at an annoying level, not very loud, but loud enough to disturb the peace. Then a nurse appears, and apologises for the time that is on my appointment letter. It is too early and I am sent away until noon. I still can't eat and can only take sips of water until 11.00am.

At noon we return and wait for another hour. I am finally admitted, but this is only the start. There is no bed for me so I sit and receive a series of visitors: the nurse who asks me questions; the radiologist who will be doing the procedure and talks me through it; the x-ray man; another nurse who cannulates me, failing painfully as he tries one hand, and succeeding equally painfully in the other. The pain is a great motivator to have the port operation, however long the fast and the wait.

At 3.00pm I walk to the operating theatre, a large room full of people and kit. I climb on to the table, trying to preserve my modesty as I am only wearing a gown, the ones that do up at the back, and non-slip socks that take me straight back to my UCLH incarceration when I put them on. The x-ray boys are standing to attention at my feet; the surgeon is on my right and another nurse on my left, ready to infuse antibiotics into the cannula and, if I scream in agony, sedation. This nurse looks old and wise and kind and a bit like Yoda. And there is another nurse who is like a studio manager, doing safety checks of everything, including me.

The health and safety nurse hooks me up to a source of oxygen with those funny tickly nostril clasps. I think of the good it's doing my brain and my complexion and breathe deeply. Then I am draped, a big blue sheet over my head so I can't watch what is going on on my right side. It would be claustrophobic but the left side is attached to the drip stand and Yoda's head appears, joining me in my blue cavern and creating a space above me, thank heavens. The surgeon's disembodied voice tells me he is giving me local anaesthetic – ouch – and some more – ouch – and then he gets going. It is just like having one of those dental procedures where you don't feel any sharp pain but you do feel the dentist is bashing you about, shoving and pulling and wrenching, only on my chest, not in my mouth. It is like being beaten up without feeling pain.

The pain, on the other hand, of the antibiotic going into the cannula is so bad that I vow I will not have sedation because that will be given the same way. Yoda is as slow and gentle as he can be, but it hurts like hell. A continuing motivation for putting up with the bashing the surgeon is giving me.

Also: no sedation now means gin and tonic later.

I am released, at last, and given a sandwich and a cup of tea at 4.30pm.

Poor Seán has been waiting in the uncomfortable waiting room all this time, but I am so glad to see him and have him help me home.

I cannot take a shower for five days.

Thursday, 13 February

Today's PET/CT scan involves radiation so I have to fast again for six hours.

I set the alarm and rise at 7.00am for my customary bowl of granola and cup of tea.

I am paying for my stacked-up invasive procedures, treating my body like a machine not a living being. I am knackered and sore and psychologically beaten up. No amount of positive thinking changes how I feel.

At 1.30pm I go to the PET clinic at St Thomas'. Seán is on day release from being my carer: this is one procedure where you are strongly encouraged not to bring anyone with you as you are made radioactive and the stuff stays around for a couple of hours afterwards. No wait today: I go straight to be weighed and measured and have my blood pressure taken, answer more questions, and then I AM CANNULATED. What?? The radiation, I am told, can't go in via the port because 'it's sticky', and a special nurse is needed to flush it with heparin to clear it afterwards. Fair enough, and in fact the port area is still very tender so I don't completely mind. Also, the nurse does the cannulation well and it goes in all right first time.

I go into the 'hot' waiting room and am given the radiation infusion through the cannula, which also doesn't hurt, thank goodness. Several of us sit or lie on beds in the hot room, waiting until the radiation has made its way around our bodies. It is dim and peaceful in here and I imagine us all gently glowing.

Then into the scanner. The nurse attempts to bind my arms to keep them still but I demur – the restraint immediately brings on claustrophobia. I promise I will keep my arms still. Last time, it was not this PET/CT scanner but the PET/MRI one that was really narrow and brought on claustrophobia. But as I slide into the scanner tube I panic. I keep completely still because I CANNOT BEAR to feel how close the tunnel is around me, I keep my eyes closed, but then I roar. 'Help! Help!' Then 'GET ME OUT OF HERE!' and I am slid upwards so my head comes out the other side, and I can breathe again.

I calm down. I say I can do this. And in I go again, clutching my hands together so hard that as I start to relax they hurt, but now I can't unclasp them because I mustn't move them. I say a Hail Mary for each finger and an Our Father for my whole body, then back to *maranatha* and I really concentrate. I keep my eyes closed. I cope. More than cope; I relax and the procedure becomes meditative.

After I am released, I go to the M & S café in the main entrance of St Thomas' and order a hot bacon roll which is the most delicious thing I have eaten for a long time. I meet D at last, the wonderful woman who told me about her stem cell transplant, whose advice and experience were so valuable at the time, and who has sent me stirring supportive texts at regular intervals ever since. It is wonderful to meet her face to face. Her story is much more dramatic than mine, and her life has demanded much, much more of her, and I am humbled and inspired all over again. She is the real deal.

We agree that we have both been enriched by our suffering and learned a lot from it that we value. But we know that we can only say that of ourselves. And we talk about good company and its importance and how our cancer has made us more confident about choosing it and not wasting energy with those who drain us.

Friday, 14 February

I am at the Cancer Centre, back in the hands of the Guy's team, no longer the responsibility of UCLH. First a meeting with the doctor, then I will have my first chemotherapy infusion of fifty-four (it doesn't seem so bad when I put it like that: eighteen cycles of three weeks on, one week off equals only fifty-four infusions). Yes it does. Fifty-four is *a lot*.

I don't have to fast but I don't enjoy the freedom not to because I don't want to overdo things with chemotherapy today. I swallow anti-sickness drugs — Domperidone and the stronger Ondansetron — and have toast and tea for breakfast.

Then to the clinic. Instead of the regular phlebotomist I have a kind young nurse to take blood from my still-sore brand new port. She is anxious about sticking a needle in it because the area is swollen and bleeding. I say it is only a little tender, which is a bit of a lie. She says the needle has to go bang in the middle of the port so, I think: You might miss? 'Deep breath.' I take a deep breath. She hits the bullseye, and then confesses she wasn't confident about doing it at all. I tell her I had full confidence in her. She says that's how she managed. Our mutual support is very sweet. She takes the blood she needs and caps off the needle so that the afternoon chemo nurses don't have to insert another one. For the rest of the morning I have a big protrusion above my right breast, all still very tender, but in a good cause: no cannulation.

The clinic's height and weight nurse likes the bright colours I'm wearing (green velvet cap, green jumper over bright red top, green trousers and bright red socks). She tells me that she used to work in a place where troubled people came to classes on socialising, and one day a lady ran the class with a heap of different coloured scarves, showing each of them which colours suited them. They brightened up as their colours were draped around them. What a difference it made. We agree that it matters immensely, and she says thank you for cheering her up when I leave her little cubicle. She cheers me up: her face shines.

Sarah receives my enormous container of twenty-four-hour urine which I had to collect in the midst of all the other procedures this week. At least collecting pee doesn't hurt. Sarah apologises as she hands me next month's enormous container. How the inconveniences of cancer treatment go on and on and on.

Thence to Dr Mary. I have to re-consent to the Cardamon trial because another side effect of Carfilzomib has emerged from the trial findings: brain damage or 'progressive multifocal leukoencephalopathy'. After an exchange about risk levels that I feel I must have, even though I am no clearer at the end of it than I was at the beginning (I think I have absolutely no chance of contracting this, but I'm not sure) I sign and am released to enter the maintenance phase of the trial. Dr Mary says that I probably wouldn't have this if I were being treated outside the trial, I would be left alone following the stem cell transplant. (Oh.) But, she says, the trend in myeloma therapy is towards longer, maintenance-style treatment, not shorter treatments with long breaks. (What? I am looking forward to freedom next year. That's why I want to get through this phase as quickly as possible.)

No one has relapsed while on maintenance in Cardamon, she says. The worst cases are still good as they maintain the myeloma levels; the best cases improve.

My test results indicate I am still in remission. (Suppose I had had the stem cell transplant and my myeloma had got worse??)

Still. Praise be.

Seán asks about the power of faith and cases of spontaneous cure. Dr Mary blinks a bit but doesn't quarrel, just says that she has never seen it, and advises eating well and keeping fit and not going on any faddish diets.

Off we go to collect my drugs. I want to take today's steroids now (I have 10mg today, 10mg tomorrow to take), so as to give myself a chance of sleeping tonight. Then I go and find F, who is also at clinic today, F who is a year ahead of me on the Cardamon trial, whose hair also fell out after the Cyclophosphamide priming for the stem cell harvest. When I see her I immediately want my hair to look like her hair. It's a bouncy, curly mop, grey but soft, while mine is very, very straight and short ('like a fruit').

At 2.30pm we are back in mothercare. It feels horribly familiar. I don't want to be here. Give me the infusion and let me go as quickly as possible.

But in spite of myself I engage. In the chair opposite me a very long, very thin man hacks and hoicks revoltingly. A small thin lady creeps back to her chair, drip stand in tow. A sweet black-haired woman bids me farewell as she leaves. A bald-headed patient, a young man, is with his most beloved by the look of it, talking quietly, heads close together, in their own world.

The port is a dream going to the lavatory with the drip. No entanglements as both my arms are free. I can feel the little cannula of the port travelling over my collarbone under my skin, which feels very strange and a bit creepy, but I love it for the pain it has prevented. And it's much better than a PICC line. Nothing like the same amount of tubing inside my body and I don't have to wear a bandage all the time so I can swim.

The infusion ends, the needle is removed from the port and a new big plaster applied. It's still rather bloody. I have to hold my top and bra away from the area for the nurse, exposing rather more chest than is modest. Mr Hacky-Hoicky and his friend stare shamelessly but I find I don't mind. No actual nipple is revealed, and if it takes Mr Hacky-Hoicky's mind off the cancer that really does seem to be ravaging his body, well and good. It stops him hacking and hoicking, at any rate. And for my part? I am bending and brothering.

Oh the endless dreary ongoingness of it all. Again, Dear Readers, I ask you: will you stay the course with me? I will try and make it exciting . . .

In the evening I start, appropriately, a jigsaw of the Sistine Chapel ceiling. It will probably take me as long as it took Michelangelo to paint the real thing. Or anyway until my maintenance treatment ends. Seán says that when a cardinal came in to look at Michelangelo's work, he asked who the big fellow with the beard in the middle of the ceiling was. Was this, then, the first time God had been depicted as a bearded man in the sky? If so, Michelangelo has a lot to answer for.

If you were to depict God, how would you do it? Most religions advise against it.

Saturday, 15 February

Today I plan a long bicycle ride or walk but it's raining and windy and probably not a good idea. Shall I go to an art gallery? Seán is in Hastings and I am in London. I don't go to an art gallery, I go shopping. I buy a teal-blue boiler suit in thick corduroy from

Anthropologie and I LOVE it. I have never been able to wear a onesie before. Never tried. My bottom is trim. Such a treat. Then I have acupuncture with the redoubtable Weidong and this settles me beautifully. I seem to be recovering from the week-long assault on my battered, wonderfully resilient body.

But the full-fat anti-emetics are giving me constipation and I think I might be getting piles. Poor trim bottom. This is not comfortable.

Fortieth Letter

Dear Readers

Sunday, 16 February

I am en route to the Community of the Resurrection, Mirfield, for a short retreat, preparation for the long months of treatment ahead. Retreat, treatment . . . the one a counterbalance to the other, both needed.

The Gospel according to St Mark ends abruptly with the empty tomb. He describes no resurrection appearances. Rather, the women who have come to dress the body are told by the angel guarding the tomb: 'He is not here . . . He is going ahead of you into Galilee' (Mark 16:6-7). If they (we) are to go to meet him, they (we) are to go into Galilee them(our)selves. The reader is left with that. I think of going to Mirfield as going to Galilee.

On arrival, I fall into the peace of the place. I read this poem, which you sent me, M, when I was still going through my kind-of-death in UCLH and which, today, finally speaks to me.

Let your mind be quiet, realising the beauty of the world
And the immense, the boundless treasures that it holds in store.
All that you have within you
All that your heart desires
All that your nature so specially fits you for −
That, or the counterpart of it
Waits embedded in the great whole, for you −
It will surely come to you.
Yet equally surely not one moment before its appointed time
    will it come.

And your crying and fever and reaching out of hands will make
  no difference.
Therefore do not begin that game at all.
Do not recklessly spill the waters of your mind in this direction
  and that,
Lest you become like a spring lost and dissipated in the desert.
But draw them together into a little compass, and hold them
  still, so still.
And let them become clear, so clear — so limpid, so mirror-like;
At last the mountains and the sky shall glass themselves in peace-
  ful beauty,
And the antelope shall descend to drink
And to gaze at his reflected image,
And the lion to quench his thirst.
And Love himself shall come and bend over
And catch his own likeness in you.[1]

I feel the words as I read them, so that my mind and my heart
quieten like the still lake, content. I have come to Galilee, now all I
need do is wait.

Monday, 17 February

I am catastrophically constipated, in wrenching pain as my bowels
move but do not open.

I resolve to sit it out. The retreat house has a lavatory block
rather than en suite bathrooms, but thankfully there are few guests,
so I remain more or less undisturbed, though I do not let myself
cry out. I am confined to the cubicle as my unwilling, wincing
sphincter lets through large and solid stools with great pain and
slowness. The minutes, then the hours, tick by. I cannot move — I
am mid-release — I am stuck to the lavatory. I want to be in church,
contemplating.

I bargain with my body.

I tell it I am sorry for all that I have put it through in the last week,
treating it as though the cancer has taught me nothing about the
need to care for it.

I tell it I am sorry for its pain, its tenderness, its tiredness, its need not to suffer anymore.

I tell it I *will* put it first.

Now, please, would it get on and evacuate?

No.

Oh, I am in so much pain. How can I have to face yet another trial like this? Surely it will come to an end? Justice demands it. I've been put through too much already.

Why, oh why, have I come to Mirfield when I should be taking care of my body at home, near a hospital, help on hand, my own bathroom by my bedroom?

I do sphincter muscle exercises learned in Pilates, twisting my body round, engaging and releasing muscles in the anal passage. I raise my knees in a squat. I think of what you said, M, that childbirth is like having a big shit. Surely, like a baby, it has to come out eventually?

The stool remains stuck.

Two hours later I stop projecting forward to the moment I will be released from my prison, and surrender to the place. I give up the idea I should be in church or doing something that looks more like what people do on retreats. This lavatory cubicle is my prayer cell now. But what is my prayer? Not mantra meditation, not quiet, still-lake waiting. I am in too much pain. I have to take extraordinary action if I am ever to leave the cubicle. This involves helping the stool be released . . . with my hand. Filthy purging is my prayer. I am revolted, but I am desperate. And the relief is unspeakable. I shower and scrub myself clean, and return to my bed to let my quivering sphincter and my quaking psyche recover.

Tuesday, 18 February

The stools are soft at last, but my sphincter has gone on strike. Once again I am in the cubicle, whimpering quietly at the pain every time a stool approaches the exit. And these stools want to leave: they churn in my gut, they hurt.

I determine to endure the pain as they pass. But it isn't enough. My sphincter simply won't respond even when I say yes, I will stand this, go forth and heave.

And I have to empty my bowel manually again. It goes on and on. And on. How can a body produce so much shit? I look at my hand, covered in my own soil. I am revolted and ashamed . . . and then I accept what is happening. What is so revolting about one's own soil? (The smell.) I work away, on and on. Finally, I can feel that I have pretty much emptied my bowel, and my profound relief confirms it. This is, truly, catharsis.

I spend a long time showering and scrubbing everything.

Then I think: do I tell you, my Dear Readers, about this? It is so very, very scatological. But yes, I will if doing so is not gratuitous. Julian writes of emptying one's 'purse full feyer', as she poetically calls the bowel, marvelling at a God who is found in the greatest and the least of our actions. And your coincidental email, J, gives me courage. You describe your own procedure with such candour, and I think 'discombobulated' is just the right word to describe how rummaging in this area makes one feel.

Is the morning's catharsis a preparation for my meeting with my beloved spiritual mentor? I take it as such. And our conversation is transcendental. She listens, and my words speak themselves into new truths. We are silent for a while. Then she responds, haltingly and with no urgency or pressure, just what presents itself to her. Our conversation gently unfolds, the universe gapes and God emerges. Yes, it is a bit like a revelatory purging. And I feel the blessing of cancer, the relishing of it, the sense that it hasn't inter-rupted my life but called me to a fuller life. One I don't need to rush towards; one that will come and find its reflection in the still lake of my soul.

Later, walking in the grounds of the monastery in the rain, I take some mud in my hands and, sitting in Br A's prayer shelter in the quiet garden, wash my hands thoroughly in it. It is a wonderful connection of my own soil and the soil of the Earth, and I don't feel revolted and separated from my body and its functions anymore, but wondrously part of the cycle of things, in the wind and rain, muddied, puddled, inwardly at peace.

Feeding and nurturing the inner being protects the outer being, goes an anonymous saying from a desert father. What feeds the inner life? Not external things, which even mindfulness or yoga can become if they are imposed as yet more tasks to add to one's list of things to do.

What will feed my inner life, these next eighteen months? I look up at the crucifix in the Calvary Garden. Christ is shamed and exposed on the cross, as I have felt shamed and exposed by my bowel experience, though no longer. I ask to be open, to stay open. I do not know who I will be after these eighteen months are over. I don't need to know now.

I am jealously guarding my attention, keeping the image of the 'lake of beauty' and its still waters in my mind as I do. All will come to you, do not rush out towards it. Patrick, my singing teacher, speaks of not trying to project the voice in singing, which dissipates its energy and robs one's breath. Sing within, let the power resonate within. Your audience will be utterly drawn to you. I still feel the fiery passion that is so much a part of my nature, but I think perhaps its power will be all the greater if it sits still within me. Not suppressed, but not flung about either.

Wednesday, 19 February

Glory be. A wet fart.

Br C has become a Dear Reader. He tells me he has decided it is spiritual reading and I am touched to my core by his humility. Br C is an old campaigner and I don't believe there is anything I can teach him. But as I learn again and again when I come here, the learning simply is, it passes between and among us, when we open ourselves to it.

Seated on a mercifully quiet train back to London, I watch the waterlogged land through which we pass, and listen to 'Gabriel's Oboe', 'Ombra Mai Fu', Schubert's 'Trout' Quintet, and other Dear Readers' music. A road winds up a hill and out of sight. I think it might be what my path is going to be like for the next leg and my heart jumps a bit with joy because it is rugged and rural and not in the least straight.

Thursday, 20 February

Question: How can you tell an extroverted physicist from an introverted physicist?
Answer: An extroverted physicist looks at your shoes when you talk to him. (Thank you, H.)

Thank you, J, for exonerating Michelangelo with a picture from the Meverell Tomb in Tideswell, dated 1462, with God the Father depicted as an old man with a beard. Michelangelo painted the Sistine Chapel ceiling a century later.

Friday, 21 February

I wake to my 'steroid alarm' – taking the dose at 6.00am in the hope that it will have worn off in time for a good night's sleep tonight. I swallow the pills with a pint of water, then remember I was meant to eat something first, so hurriedly swallow a banana too.

I will not indulge in full-fat anti-emetic high dose Ondansetron unless I have to. This week I will just take Domperidone, today and tomorrow.

Waiting to check in with the receptionist for my chemotherapy, I observe with distaste the terrible behaviour of two ladies in front of me, one a patient, the other her companion. She is a private patient but says she has been sent down here – so demeaning (she doesn't say that, but she looks it) – for her chemotherapy. The receptionist can find no record of her appointment on his system. The women are sharp-tongued, critical, pushy, will not budge despite his helplessness. Eventually they submit, with little grace, returning upstairs to the grandly carpeted private care 'village' to give someone else hell. Naturally they are anxious; we all are. Last week I had been hard on the radiology nurse who came to tell me that my port operation would be delayed by some hours. Seán said to me then, we should be unfailingly kind. The glitches are not the fault of the messenger.

In the waiting area loud voices irritate and disturb my peace. I am editing. But I bend and brother and interosculate and the sounds soften, flowing into and around me, and I am able to concentrate once more on my task.

The port plaster comes off. The scar is healing well. But the thing makes quite a bump and there'll be no sequin boob tubes worn by me this year.

En route to Hastings I feel nauseous and swallow one lower-dose Ondansetron pill. Fingers crossed. I am caught between the Scylla of nausea and the Charybdis of constipation. I want to eat plain white food but that — white bread, white rice, white everything — is going to gum me up.

Forty-first Letter

Dear Readers

Wednesday, 26 February

I go to midday eucharist to have my forehead ashed at St George the Martyr. 'Remember that dust thou art, and to dust thou wilt return,' the priest intones, as he marks us with a cross made of ash and oil. And so Lent begins, a period of fasting, praying, almsgiving and repentance.

I *namaste* everyone at the peace, hurriedly explaining about the chemotherapy because they are all shaking hands with each other and I don't want them to think I'm a coronavirus wuss. The priest recommends not intincting the wafer but drinking from the common cup. This doesn't make sense to me, so I just don't drink from the cup.

E.O. Wilson warned that we are entering the Eremezoic Era: the era of loneliness, as the planet becomes more unhealthy and we have to secure ourselves against poisonous air, water and soil. We may also have to secure ourselves against each other.

I head to the King's Road to John Sandoe's bookshop to pick up *Jumpers* by Tom Stoppard, which I need for a reference. *Upstream*, essays by Mary Oliver, catches my eye and demands to be bought as well. Poetic and stirring, the essays are all about connectedness.

And then I find the most delicious pair of khaki baggy pantaloons by Toast in Peter Jones. In them I would not look out of place among the pastoralia on stage at the Globe.

Thence to my fabulous hairdresser Judith and I am emotional, again, because she snips at my crop, applies some wax, muddles it a bit and combs it and applies the hairdryer, and I REALLY LIKE what I see. It's still a bit short but it's a great thatch of hair. My leftover hair – the Al shrive – was silvery, a bit like my oldest brother's hair, only I had less of it than he has. My new hair is like my next older brother's hair, a thick thatch, possibly wavy, I can't tell yet, not ginger like his but the same texture.

My hair has its first outing to the Boot and Flogger with L, who is so encouraging: 'Not cancer hair. New Claire hair.'

Thursday, 27 February

Skipping back to the flat along Borough High Street, high on George Herbert's poetry I've just heard at Southwark Cathedral, I decide I can't wait until the wax Judith has recommended has arrived in the post and go into Sainsbury's. I find something that resembles what she applied, but it is for men, and it is called 'clay'. There's another tin of similar-looking substance for men and it's called 'putty'. Women's hair gunk would never be called that, would it? Do names like clay and putty make the application of wax, for appearance, seem more manly and gruff, not like a girl?

As I rub the 'clay' into my hair in my bathroom I remember the mud on my hands in Mirfield, and I feel I am interosculating with nature.

Friday, 28 February

I ask my chemotherapy nurse what the protocol is for coronavirus. She says that if someone turns up in the chemotherapy suite with flu-like symptoms they are to be put immediately in an isolation room, the door closed, and left alone to phone 111. Meanwhile everyone whom they have been near has to be contacted: that's everyone in the reception area, everyone who might have been in a lift with them, and all the patients and staff in the chemotherapy suite. And all of these people have to phone 111, and then possibly go into quarantine. Cancer patients have compromised immune systems so we are really vulnerable. I ask why we aren't all given huge pieces of red paper with the message written on them: If you feel ill

STAY AT HOME, you buggers, because you will cause untold havoc and trouble if you start mixing with other people in the Cancer Centre.

Saturday, 29 February

What fabulous responses you have sent to last week's scatological confessions. A ton of advice: strong black coffee with lots of sugar; kiwi fruit; non-alcoholic beer; glycerine pessaries. And thanks to lovely attentive nurse Grace, a prescription for lashings of laxatives. And this (thank you, L):

> We read of blessed Gregory that while he was purging his bowels and saying a psalm, the devil appeared to him and asked him what he was doing. He responded, 'I am purging my bowels and praising my God', since works of nature are not seen as turpid to the perfect.[2]

And the famous *Spitting Image* sketch about the Queen's bottom, dear H, from the 1980s:

Prince Andrew: So, how was New Zealand, Ma?
Queen: Super! We saw ever so many interesting factories, didn't we Philip? And lots of bottoms.
A: Gosh, wizard!
Q: Yes, I must say, the bottoms were splendid.
A: I didn't think you'd like the bottoms, Mater.
Q: Oh no, they were super.
Prince Philip: She doesn't know what a bottom is.
Q: I can't think why we don't have them over here.
A: Oh Ma!
Q: Well I'm the Queen and I want bottoms in Britain.
P: You silly old picnic rug, we've all got bottoms in Britain.
Q: I haven't.
P: You have, you have. I've told you a million times you've got one.
Q: No I haven't.

A: Yes you have, Ma. I mean, what about when you go to the loo?

Q: I don't go to the loo. I'm the Queen.

A: Mater, when you sit down, what is it you sit down on?

Q: Cushions.

A: But what's on the cushion?

Q: The Queen, obviously.

A: Under the Queen?

Q: The throne.

A: And?

Q: My subjects.[3]

And I have to believe, S, you former drag queen you, that you were once in a punk band called Manual Evacuation.

Now on this chemotherapy sabbath I am trying to eat food that is not constipation-inducing as well as not being nausea-inducing. White toast and white rice are out. Pears are in, and porridge, egg, avocado, cooked lettuce (not all at once). Thank heavens I am not so nauseous this time that I can't face green food. But even though I have had no Ondansetron at all, and I'm eating sensibly, I'm still constipated. It must be psychological. Thanks to you, I am now surrounded by remedies.

Forty-second Letter

Dear Readers

Sunday, 1 March

It hits me again (does one ever get used to this?) that I will have cancer for the rest of my life, even if I am lucky enough to stay in remission for lengthy periods. It's as though there's something in me that *will* keep on denying my mortality, like a default setting: I cannot bear too much reality. I breathe, receive again the knowledge of my mortality, accept it, turn it to good use: making art of my life. Do not delay what has to be done, but pace yourself. And find joy today. This is not just how to live with cancer; it's how to live.

Thank you, G, for sending this:

> No heaven can come to us
> Unless our hearts find rest in today.
> Take Heaven!
> No peace lies in the future which is not
> Hidden in this present moment.
> Take Peace!
> The gloom of the world is but a shadow.
> Behind it, yet within our reach, is joy.
> Take Joy!
> Life is so full of meaning and purpose, so full
> of beauty that you will find earth but
> cloaks your heaven. Courage then to claim it.
> That is all.[4]

251

I should not try to do everything now, cramming things in, slotting them together with no thought for my body's need to pace itself more naturally, and my mind's need for tranquility and adequate preparation. Irish J says: 'pressure is for tyres'. This is a journey to relish.

Today I read and recognise this thought from Mary Oliver in *Upstream*: 'I saw the difference between doing nothing, or doing a little, and the redemptive act of true effort. Reading, then writing, then desiring to write well, shaped in me that most joyful of circumstances — a passion for work.'[5]

Monday, 2nd March

Given a Pilates exercise which ends up in a shoulder stand, I try to get to the shoulder stand instead of properly engaging the internal sacral transverse corset, the gluteous muscles of my bottom, and pulling in my tummy and letting all those muscles pull my legs up. Once I stop trying to get to the finishing line and just concentrate on the muscles I need, it happens.

I am reading a book for review and have tasked myself with finishing it today so the review can be written tomorrow. I skim read, not enjoying it, not relishing the arguments, losing interest in the task. I stop myself, reset, drop the notion of finishing and determine to enjoy reading. I have to trust there will be time to do what is needful. Now the book is finishing itself and it's quite good.

I am to go back to Westminster Abbey this week and I am anxious. I remind myself of how much I love my colleagues and my work. I will dissipate my anxiety by remembering to enjoy myself.

Tuesday, 3 March

The ride is somehow right in every way. I am on Denby, and he feels lighter, less like a solid mountain, more like a fluid thing, a deep-running river perhaps, that always holds the possibility of becoming rapids and can never be taken for granted, but whose flow I can enter and be carried by.

You say it must all be happening down my way, dear C, and it is. Maybe e e cummings is right about spring being 'perhaps' at the start, as the snowdrops then crocuses and primroses poke their heads above ground and open up to the sometimes-sun and the sky: they are there but tentative, because there may well be more frost and coldness to destroy their bold uprightness and the bright splashes of white and pink and purple and yellow. But then nature explodes, and there is nothing 'perhaps' about her fecundity. It is just wonderful to look at all of this, and the muddy ground and the budding hedgerow and the three buzzards hovering over the copse, from the back of a horse.

The book review gets written.

Friday, 6 March

This is my week off chemotherapy but I have to go to Guy's today to have my teeth checked before I restart Zometa, the bone-strengthening bisphosphonate. The lovely dentist uses a great phrase in relation to the molar that is still sensitive since the stem cell transplant. It's the 'first tooth standing'. I think: one day in decrepitude we'll have the 'last tooth standing'. The 'left' and 'right' of our teeth are called from the point of view of the patient, not the dentist, just like stage directions. 'Stage right, first tooth standing.'

I am wearing my teal corduroy boiler suit, pearls and my punky hair. I feel a bit like a glam plumber.

Waiting for an x-ray of my teeth I am distressed by many of my fellow patients' stature. Stooped and crabbed and stiff-jointed. I want to lead a Pilates session here, now.

One lady in a bright yellow shirt is hot and clearly suffering. I have been irritated by an apparent increase in the frequency of my hot flushes, waking me hourly at night and making me uncomfortable during the day. But this dear lady is *dripping*. Her distress silences my grumbles at my less troublesome lot. Discomfort is not nearly a strong enough word for what she is suffering, but hot flushes are not painful, so what is the word?

Thank you, J, for the even earlier, much earlier, reference to God as an old man, in Daniel 7:9, which declares that the Ancient of Days has hair as white as wool and he sits on a throne. He doesn't have a beard though.

Week four: I am at the end of my first maintenance chemotherapy cycle. One down. Seventeen to go. Seventeen.

Saturday, 7 March

I think my hair is now looking a bit smug. Sensible. I don't really want to be or look those things. But it's growing all the time.

Sunday, 8 March

Today is the anniversary of my diagnosis, as you noticed, lovely J! What a distance we've come this year, my dear friends all. How fantastic it has been to have your company and what a difference you have made to the experience. I can't thank you enough.

A year of being a person living with cancer, the first year of the rest of my life with my till-death-do-us-part myeloma. I *will* put it to work: it will motivate me to make who I am a work of art, and these are the qualities I shall cultivate: 'imaginative energy, radiance, equilibrium, composure, colour, light, vitality, poise, buoyancy, a transcendent ability to soar above life and not be subjugated by it'.[6]

Thus, death will have no dominion.

Forty-third Letter

Dear Readers

Instead of shaking hands at the exchange of peace at church, we *namaste* each other, quite naturally. Brilliant interfaith wisdom. And although the reason isn't good, it's a relief not to be the only one being careful now.

You write, dear JF: 'If living like horses means living each moment seamlessly flowing from one moment to the next, negating the need to have expectations as to what to expect of the next moment, it occurred to me that you and Seán may be doing just that in your present lives . . . all the while forming bonds with people and beings.'
  Thank you.

Tonight I restart my 5.30–6.30pm silent time in church. I take Julian with me but it is too dark to read her, so instead I recall to mind her seventh revelation in which she speaks of experiencing a deep, wonderful joy, swiftly replaced by an equally deep loss of comfort and ease, then the joy again, then the dis-ease, back and forth, some twenty times. Weal and woe: we will suffer them both. Then I sink gladly into depth and silence of my own. The place feeds my thirsty soul.

Tuesday, 10 March

I ride sinuous L'Arcelle in a gentle hack around the less waterlogged paths and lanes of the farm. Mist descends. Do I see hawthorn emerging? I must check my almanac (thank you, A) for what to expect in the hedgerows this month.

Wednesday, 11 March

I am back in my office in Westminster Abbey at last, and loving it. I don't even mind my colleagues' double takes as my head is now exposed with its thatch of charcoal grey. Their responses are so genuinely warm and welcoming. And my shorn head is evidence of my trials. I wouldn't want anyone to think I'd been skiving.

Thursday, 12 March

The pictures we are being shown, a lot, of the coronavirus with its coat of fatty suckers that need twenty seconds of scrubbing in hot soapy water to be dispelled, remind me of a wonderful project. A woman was flicking through a Sunday paper magazine and suddenly, upon seeing an image, experienced a really nasty physical reaction. It turned out that what she had seen was an image of a virus that had previously attacked her body, making her ill. Somehow, just seeing it had provoked a response. This gave her boyfriend an idea. If we are hurt by looking at viruses that can cause disease, would we be helped by looking at viruses or other vectors that have good effects? He looked up images for the hormones and neurotransmitters that are released when we fall in love. The images of these are beautiful and he created a 'love logo' from a skilful artistic combination of them. Meanwhile, now, I find myself averting my eyes from images of the coronavirus.

I go to evensong, exquisitely sung by the Lay Vicars. Although I love the choristers, hearing the men on their own always makes me think of how the Abbey must have sounded pre-Reformation, when the monks chanted their endless psalms of praise and repentance and thanksgiving. I feel as though I have come home again. And I love the Lenten prayer of penitence:

Almighty and everlasting God, who hatest nothing that thou hast made and dost forgive the sins of all them that are penitent: Create and make in us new and contrite hearts, that we, worthily lamenting our sins and acknowledging our wretchedness, may obtain of thee, the God of all mercy, perfect remission and forgiveness; through Jesus Christ our Lord. Amen.[7]

Friday, 13 March

At the clinic I am given a sobering talk by Sarah, followed up by the doctor: the latest coronavirus guidance for cancer patients puts me on the high-risk register. I tick three boxes: I am receiving immuno-suppressive chemotherapy; I have had a stem cell transplant; and I have myeloma, which is one of the riskier cancers.

Seán is also at risk. He and I should refrain from all but necessary social interaction in crowded places. But what counts as necessary? I regard evensong as necessary; the Fellows' Programme as necessary; one-to-one encounters at work; Pilates; horse riding; all as necessary. And I am bursting to get on with things now I am back at the Abbey. The doctor is only adamant about avoiding crowds and leaves the rest to our discretion, but she is grave.

I return in the afternoon for my infusions of Carfilzomib and Zometa. The chemotherapy nurses are being driven mad, though you would not know it, by the laboratory's lengthy delay preparing our various chemotherapies; by the computer system crashing across the hospital site, so none of our drug prescriptions can be ordered, let alone collected and delivered to us; and by difficult patients like me who insist that I am owed some more steroids. I am wrong and I waste nurse Andy's time but he does not cease to speak in a quiet, kind voice though his eyes are tired and he has been on the go for hours. God bless these nurses who will all be late finishing tonight.

When we finally emerge from the hospital it is rush hour, so we go back to the flat and wait to catch a later, quieter train. But how busy is rush hour anyway? How busy will it be next week? The news is getting worse by the moment.

The spirit is a garden and prayer is gardening, says Victor Hugo.

I am under the weather. Chemotherapy sabbath! I did not sleep much at all last night, nor had I the night before. I have a kind of low-level running nausea, not bad enough to warrant strong anti-emetics — I now have a different one from the constipation-inducing Ondansetron — but horrid nevertheless, and I am tired. In the night I worry, irrationally, about the Institute. Sleepless nights are much more bearable if I'm not worried about anything. I just read until I feel sleepy again. Now, as I toss and turn, I think: I will write to my colleagues. Then they can worry, and I can sleep.

Mrs Cohen is woken by Mr Cohen, who is tossing and turning and moaning. She asks him what is wrong. He tells her he owes Goldberg 250 shekels and can't pay him. Mrs Cohen goes to the window, raises it, and calls across the street: 'Mr Goldberg! Mr Goldberg!' Eventually Goldberg comes to his window, bleary eyed. 'Yes?' Mrs Cohen says: 'You know my husband owes you 250 shekels?' 'Yes?' says Goldberg. 'Well he can't pay you,' says Mrs Cohen. Then she slams the window shut and comes back to bed. 'You can sleep,' she says to her husband. 'Now Goldberg is the one who's awake worrying about your debt.'

I wake and I am much better. I have slept, I have an appetite, and I have energy. And I am deeply grateful for these gifts because I have briefly been denied them.

The papers are full of warnings and Seán and I discuss what we might do as things unfold. We may both be required to self-isolate, but where: London or Hastings (oh, how lucky to have the choice)? Do we need to be near our hospitals and our drug suppliers? Will hospitals be places to avoid at all costs (will my maintenance chemo-therapy cease)? Is London better because facilities are closer; or Hastings because the air is cleaner, the views from Sunbeam's windows are expansive and we won't get cabin fever?

We cannot be complacent. But we've not been complacent all year: we've had a bit more time than most to practise living with our vulnerable mortality.

Forty-fourth Letter

Dear Readers

There is nothing special about my situation now; my new normal is everyone's new normal.

But I want to be a leader in this global pandemic, not a measly weakling stuck at home whose only service is not to get ill. I want to be up and at it. I've been weak ALL YEAR. I've surrendered enough. I want to update my status, become a hero on a journey again, not to be silent waiting at home.

My shoulders are concrete-tense and it takes a lot of work even to begin to exercise properly in Pilates, where the primary task today, and often, is to move the generation of energy in each exercise from the shoulders and neck to the abdomen where the really powerful muscles are. Pilates mainly shows up my off-balanced state, but I persevere in moving my attention from my mind to my body and imaginatively to the muscles I want to awaken, and something shifts. Anyway, walking back I am able to breathe the sea air and blink at the sun, and not hurry into unknown worries. I can pace myself.

Glenda leaves us with a task, to keep imagining we are holding an orange between our shoulder blades. Goodness it makes a difference, if only to show how hunched I become as I walk anxiously from place to place.

Meditating in church, I consciously invite porosity to pierce holes in the granite of my being that is still trying to hold up the world like Atlas; softening and receiving and responding, not doing and fighting. I'm being called to something deeper and quieter. I'm tussling

259

with a feeling of letting the Abbey down. I'm trying to accept this new way of being, which is transformative and the transformation is not just for me. Gradually I stop listening to my breath, I stop repeating *maranatha*. I simply, deeply, rest in God, like Julian's beholding, a deep one-ing of my soul with God, God alone, God Godself.

My laptop charger had failed, sending me into a panic, but when I get back I twiddle it a bit and it is working again. But the lead is clearly fraying – all that travelling back and forth between Hastings and London – and I order two more, praying I've ordered the right ones. The other deeply awful thing about ordering online, apart from the endless attention pestering, is that you don't know whether the picture of the thing you want on the screen is actually the thing you want. Unless you have it in your hands, how do you know? This is something I am clearly going to have to get over in the coming weeks.

To deal with the threat of coronavirus we have to disconnect physically, stop touching, or 'touch only with our eyes' as the Maldivian scuba diving instructors taught us of our excursions into the underwater seascape of the Indian Ocean. Our transformations and connections and kindlings of love come, often, from face-to-face encounter, when we feel our porosity to each other, when it becomes evident. The challenge is not to disconnect. Thank God for technology, but thank God even more for our imaginations, our empathy, our focused attention, our love, into the service of which technology has to be brought.

And indeed messages of support and offers of help to neighbours are pouring in through my 'Nextdoor Borough' email feed. Gentleness is soaking upwards from the deep.

Thank God for bidets. We are nervous about returning to London – well I am – for a number of reasons, one significant one being that in my flat I am down to three loo rolls and I have no bidet. Have bidet: use much, much less loo roll. We have two here at the house in Hastings – and a lot of loo rolls besides.

I look up the almanac to find out what will be growing in the hedge-row in March. I probably saw blackthorn, not hawthorn, bud-bursting last week. I find I can also look for pussy-willow catkins, sweet violet, three-cornered garlic, primrose and wood anemone: 'In every bud: the coiled spring' (thank you, I).[8]

This evening we rebel and go to the FILO for a pint. It is subdued and half empty so we are able to keep our six feet distance; but there is so much touching! Glasses, the chair, the table, the loo . . . It is a delicious pint and lovely to see Sam the barman, who shows me his sore hands, chapped from so much washing, and to catch up with Mike the owner, but we shouldn't have done it.

In the fish and chip shop we hear vox pop. Boris is not loved. 'He's made a fucking mess of it,' asserts a man, admittedly drunk. 'It's all right for him, he's not going to lose his job.'

Tuesday, 17 March

Nature is waking up but the sky holds its breath. The air is still. It is St Patrick's Day. My mother's birthday, God rest her. Seán's and my anniversary of becoming a couple.

My heart breaks a little as N and I agree we should not go riding. Rachel sends a lovely kind message from the stables. I feel foolish as I ask her to look after the horses — well, yes, Claire, I think we can manage that — but I want to tell my thanks for the way they have kept me sane and on the road to recovery for a year. As I write this, tears are pouring down my face. Some things are hard to give up. I shan't be looking for the 'coiled spring' in blackthorn buds in the hedgerow from horseback this year.

I am off balance. Profoundly anxious, shaken, lost. Unable to settle. I need to settle, not to add to the noise of it all, I must be one of those who has to stay safe and away. I'm not on a planning committee or a leadership team. Just trying to stay steady and not cause trouble.

We may have theoretical visions of the kind of society we want to be and work politically or with activism towards it, but we are, in practice, forged on events like this. Will we learn to live more slowly?

Back in London, I shop. So much touching. I wear gloves but forget what I've touched with my gloves and what I've touched with my bare hands. No loo rolls to be had, even for ready money, in Borough High Street.

Wednesday, 18 March

In the night I lie awake, listening to the occasional lorry roar along Marshalsea Road, bringing loo rolls, I hope. A blackbird warbles. It's 3.50am.

I throw myself into the hands of the living God.

It is morning and I am scared. I am doing a codeword puzzle and trying to concentrate my mind. And I find I am drawing on the Blitz spirit. I just am. It's there in me, it's part of our story. It braces me, wakes up a brisk, no-nonsense attitude for which I am grateful, but I'm also chastened. I thought we needed to lay to rest our Second World War myth because the story we need now is not battle but quest, to deal with the ecological crisis. I think I'm right about needing not to think of our twenty-first-century challenges, including this virus, as battles, but we need the Blitz spirit and it is here, in us.

I learn that the ban on lorries driving through London between 9.00pm and 4.00am has been lifted, so they can bring supplies to our shops. JF is sent foraging for loo roll and finds some.

Survival of the fittest is not the principle at work now, not for humanity, even if nature is picking off the weakest by means of the virus. We are doing what we can to protect the vulnerable. This is what humans are made of. Deep kindness. Offers are flooding in to me, not least from you, Dear Readers. We are in this together and, like the 'prisoners' dilemma',[9] we will only manage it if we all work together.

Thursday, 19 March

I worry about interior suffering. We can't gather to dispel our fears. Thank God for digital technology, thank God. But there will be all sorts of hidden horrors or just sheer frustration, boredom, unhappiness, depression going on indoors. And also great strengths discovered. Lord, I pray for those to be magnified in every human in every way.

The *Today* programme is thankfully restored to its rightful place of sensible reporting and comment, on which Secretaries of State are once again appearing. It's already hard to remember the hissy disdain of ministers refusing to be interviewed. And this morning Gordon Brown speaks about what he learned from his experience of the 2008 global financial crisis. He says: 'No more America first, India first, China first.' The health challenges of coronavirus and their economic fallout have to be met globally.

The programme finishes with an opera singer lifting our spirits. She can't sing on stage so this is a bit of work for her, and a bit of joy for us. We will hear from an artist like this every day.

The new chargers for my laptop arrive. I am saved, as I tell the delivery man, thanking him profusely for his service. And they are the right ones. Glory be.

A long cycle to Rotherhithe along the Thames. Empty streets, quiet river, open pubs, not busy. I love this old town, I adore its majestic river.

I return to a message from the Cancer Centre: we are asking you not to bring a companion with you, to minimise human traffic. So I am expected: my treatment is continuing, for now.

5.00pm. I cough. Twice. A dry cough. And then half an hour later I cough again. I take my temperature. It's normal, but panic shoots like a warning cannonball across my bows. If I've contracted the virus — if I have just one of the two symptoms — I am in isolation and have to stay here at the flat. No treatment tomorrow, no train to Hastings. Fear rises like a great wave, and washes over me and passes on. I recover my balance. But the shock jolts me into empathy for the panic buyers. And for those who suddenly become prisoners or refugees, fleeing with no time to plan what to take, what to leave. You become quite animal-like. You cannot think straight. Your decisions are crazy.

So you have to wait for the wave to pass, even if you don't have much time. You have to wait, and breathe. Feel the wave pass. Then see what 'necessary' means. What can I not do without?

Friday, 20 March

I don't cough again and my temperature remains normal.

The Abbey is now closed and all staff are to stay and work at home. So much for my plans. The Dean writes: 'I do not do this lightly. I want you to know that the clergy will keep the services going as they should. We intend to have things to say and share, and we will keep the building loved and safe, so that we can step back into it together when this is over. I will miss you. We will pray for you.'

There is a little coffee shop just across the road from my flat. People in there are standing closer than six feet, but looking very serious and ignoring each other, as if they would be kept safe by disconnecting psychologically rather than physically. I understand this: my experience of putting on a mask after chemotherapy made the whole world 'other' as if there were an invisible shield around me; I was alien. Not catching anyone's eye made me feel spuriously safe from a world that seemed poisonous.

We have to be counter-intuitive. Stand six feet away, yes, but smile, and talk. Connect with our eyes, our laughter and our words.

I walk to the Cancer Centre. We pedestrians practise wide berth walking. Some shrink away as if that will protect them as well as distance; others smile across the gap and exude warmth.

I am met by a phalanx of volunteers at the door. You may not pass until you have answered questions about your health, says the Ewbank-eyelashed lady to me, and (they are still working out the system) "Give her a piece of paper: we have to have her piece of paper,' the receptionist to the volunteer. 'Give me some paper to give her, then,' she replies, her eyelashes and her face entirely unruffled. I duly receive my chit and am checked in by a member of staff. No touch screens today, hurray! Up in the lift: we clumsily hit the buttons with our elbows.

I am among matter-of-fact heroes. The nurses, many of them my friends now, Deniz and Vicky and Jing, in a laughing not-too-close huddle making plans for the day.

The patient opposite me is feverishly washing her hands, helping herself to the nurses' gloves, wrapping herself in masks and tissue and heaven knows what else. She is really scared. We do some deep breathing together. We become friends.

The auxiliary nurse comes to check 'me vitals'. She is a scary mother who tells me about her sixteen-year-old son. He heard her cough yesterday, he was upstairs and she was in the living room, a cough caused by drinking some water which went down the wrong way. He shouts to her to stay where she is; she has to self-isolate in the living room and stay there. He will cook dinner. He does, and he cleans the bathroom. She tells me, laughing, 'I said you've got to keep this up for a year, son.'

The embrace-from-a-distance which I did not see in the coffee shop is certainly happening here, waiting outside mothercare to be called for my treatment. We weakling cancer patients are leaders in the new field of Covid-safe communion. We sit distributed around the foyer, smiling at each other and leaving each other in our own peace. Then the lady sitting nearest me tells me about her friend trying to buy her food at Lidl in Greenford. Three fights broke out. The vulnerable group was allowed in first and I had insensitive images of ninety-year-olds bashing each other with their sticks and Zimmer frames, but they were behaving, she said. The fights were among the youngsters in the queue outside. Her daughter who is pregnant went to go ahead of the queue and was accosted by a man who questioned her pregnant status. He said, I have three children. It's hard.

She has skin cancer and shows me truly revolting pictures of her red, scabby scalp with some pride, beating me hands down in the symptoms competition.

For my infusion I am again seated opposite masked-up M, my new friend. She tries to drink without taking off her mask, sliding a straw round and behind it into her mouth. The nurses tease her and she relaxes. Her attempts to keep the world at bay with her masks and tissues look like the forlorn and useless coastal defences against rising seas. This is nature who is up and at us, not other people. Nature. Nature will prevail. We have to learn to live with her, not fight her, just as I have had to learn to live with, actually love, my cancer. It is a default setting, to talk about winning the fight against the coronavirus, and will do for now, but only for now: nature will not be stopped or defeated (come to think of it, does anyone ever, truly win a war?).

I am in admiration of and fascinated by the way we are adjusting, how people of goodwill are seeking the best responses and changing as we learn more. The systems are tripping over themselves to respond aright in the light of scientific developments. We must cut our government some slack, trying to make decisions and give clear advice when reliable information is still so scarce.

The man immediately opposite me looks default miserable. I catch his eye and he closes them. I don't know if he is embarrassed or cross. His mouth is set in a downwards drag of discontent. I think he's probably quite jolly somewhere inside and I will try to elicit a smile before I leave. Now he is being lovely with nurse Vicky. Oh, he's pulling his trousers down. No, just exposing his tummy for an injection. It looks so sore, and now we are smiling at each other and he explains he's been having his chemotherapy through his tummy for a year now and every time it starts to feel less sore he has to have some more. He's a complete sweetie. I wonder what my face looks like in repose??

My treatment over, I leave Guy's, cross the road, and clamber straight on to a train at London Bridge. It is right to be leaving London, though I don't like deserting my beloved old city. The journey is so easy, I will only have to come back once a week for treatment, and I can choose trains carefully. This one has some passengers, but we can easily sit six feet apart from each other, and we do. Many of us have suitcases. Fleeing the danger.

At my seat I look out of the window at the passing countryside, nearly empty of humans. Two people, one dog, in one enormous playing field.

Saturday, 21 March

Some of these thoughts are inspired by Anthony Selden's comments today on *The Week in Westminster.*

What happens to 'teach to the test' when the tests aren't going to take place? What is teaching for, then? Can we re-envision education, having been forced to drop our algorithmised counting of children's box-ticking? Can we kindle and feed the love of learning in our young people? Teach them focused attention and resilience? Give them good company and teach them how to be good company themselves? Set aside their fear of failure and dare to take risks?

When my diary empties and I can no longer judge my status and that of others by how busy we all are, when we are all in that same position, what is my time then for? I no longer have the excuse of not having time to think what my life is; I have time, and I can think, imagine, dream, confront, deepen, really, really question and answer honestly. Take time to know myself better, find out what I love, give myself to that. I've had some practice, this last year.

When I cannot do the one thing most humans naturally do in times of trouble, which is to physically congregate and commune, how do I overcome the obstacles to connection? We know how critical communion is to health, and not just human health; many other animals suffer from isolation, like the caged sows I heard about on *Farming Today*. We can get out in the fresh air, and stand six feet apart from each other, and smile so warmly that the day changes for both of us. (Though shouting can be annoying. Walking down Croft Road to the shop for some teabags, I met three neighbours in a row and had three lovely, probably quite loud, chats. A lady came out of her front door and looked at me disparagingly.) These are encounters that have to mean something quite quickly because we don't have the luxury of an evening together letting our diffident souls be softened by wine. You can stand six feet apart in a queue and talk about standing six feet apart in a queue, in a soothing or lively or funny way. The Blitz spirit at a distance. Encounters are with strangers who can become friends. We practise this at chemotherapy. Just be warm and loving. It's actually much less threatening to both parties when you're too far apart to have to worry about unwanted intimacy.

Technology is a means to an end, not an end in itself. So what is the end it should serve? We have time to explore that question, and put ourselves in charge of it again. We humans, not algorithms, can know our real needs. Our real, deep needs are the ends technology should serve. What are they?

Sunday, 22 March

I read on the Myeloma UK website that in the next few days I will be advised to self-isolate for twelve weeks.

So Be It.

Here's my prayer of preparation:

> GOD!!!!
> Help me to let the waves of fear pass over and away.
> Help me to be porous, not prickly, with the universe.
> Help me to practise what quietens my mind; what gener-
> ates energy; what makes me laugh; what helps me
> sleep.
> Help me to think of a good, disciplined way to spend
> time online.
> Help me prepare my stubborn soul to ask for help (I
> really need help with this).
> Help me to understand I am helping just by staying safe.
> Amen.

As I write the prayer, my heart falters and tears fall. So many more miles to go. How will I bear it?

Like this: I put on some lipstick, straighten my shoulders, open my heart, and walk towards the next challenge.

Dear Readers' Playlist

Abba, 'Dancing Queen' (M)
Allegri, 'Miserere Mei' (A and C)
Aurora, 'Apple Tree' (Georgia Remix) (W)
Joan Armatrading, 'Love and Affection' (C)
Louis Armstrong, 'It's a Wonderful World' (C)
Ascension, 'Beauty in All Things' (L)

Bach, *Goldberg Variations* (U)
Bach, Partita in B Flat (played by Dinu Lipatti) (P)
Bach, Double Violin Concerto (P)
Bach, 'Jesu, meiner Freude' (V)
Beatles, 'Here Comes the Sun' (J)
Beatles, 'Something' (I)
Beatles, 'I Wanna Hold Your Hand' (P)
Beethoven, 'Cavatina' (M)
Beethoven, Piano Sonatas 30, 31 and 32 (played by John Lill) (P)
Beethoven, Quartet No. 14 in C Sharp Minor, Opus 131 (P)
Andrea Bocelli, 'Nelle Tue Mani' (A)
Brahms, *Requiem*, soprano solo, fifth movement (T)
Brahms, Violin Concerto (P)
Brahms, Symphony No. 2, first movement (Leonard Bernstein and Vienna Philharmonic) (D)
Brahms, 'Academic Festival Overture', Opus 80 (B)
Dave Brubeck, 'Strange Meadow Lark' (A)
Sarah Blasko, 'All I Want' (I)
Jeff Buckley, 'Hallelujah' (P)
William Byrd, 'Descendit de Caelis' (Cardinall's Musick) (P)
Jacques Brel, 'Le Plat Pays qui est le Mien' (M)
Billy Bragg, 'Jerusalem' (S)
Bax, 'Mater, ora filium' (C)
Bizet, 'Pearl Fishers Duet' (C)

Thomas Campion, 'Never Weather-beaten Sail' (sung by Alfred Deller) (P)
Pablo Casals, 'The Song of the Birds' (T)
Mama Cass, 'Make Your Own Kind of Music' (S)

Chopin, Polonaise in A Flat Major (S)
Chopin, Nocturne in D Flat, Opus 27, No. 2 (played by Lang Lang) (A)
Chopin, Prelude in E Minor (R)
Petula Clark, 'Don't Sleep in the Subway' (M)
College and Electric Youth, 'A Real Hero' (J)
Eva Cassidy, *Songbird* (L)
Eva Cassidy, 'Over the Rainbow' (L)
Leonard Cohen, 'Alleluia' (E)
Leonard Cohen, 'You Want it Darker' (C)

Debussy, 'Clair de Lune' (A)
Delius, *Sea Drift* (sung by Bryn Terfel) (A)
Desire, 'Under Your Spell' (J)

Elgar, 'Where Corals Lie' (L)
Elgar, *The Dream of Gerontius* (M and T)
Elgar, *The Kingdom* (S)
Elisa, 'Almeno Tu Nell'Universo' (V)
Everything But the Girl, 'Missing' (L)

Fauré, 'Cantique de Jean Racine' (F and J)
Kathleen Ferrier, 'The Keel Row' (L)
Kathleen Ferrier, 'Blow the Wind Southerly' (M)
Fifth Dimension, 'Wedding Bell Blues' (J)
Finzi, 'Dies Natalis' (G)
Finzi, Clarinet Concerto (G)
Fireball XL5 theme tune (M)
The Five Stairsteps, 'Oooh Child' (L)
Ella Fitzgerald, 'Summertime' (A)
Ella Fitzgerald, 'Every Time We Say Goodbye' (P)

Jan Garbarek, *Officium* (C and I)
Philip Glass, *Passages* (C)
Philip Glass, *Satyagraha* (L)
The Gloaming, 'Rolling Wave' (P)
Gluck, 'Che Faro Senza Euridice' (both Kathleen Ferrier's and Janet Baker's) (P)
Charlie Gracie, 'Wandering Eyes' (M)
David Gray, 'Please Forgive Me' (L)
Norman Greenbaum, 'Spirit in the Sky' (L)
Gregorian Chants, 'Inno: Conditor', 'Pater Noster' and 'Agnus Dei' (A)
Grieg, Piano Concerto in A Minor (R)
Nacha Guevara, 'La Noche' (T)

Handel, 'Ombra Mai Fu' (M)
Handel, 'Hallelujah Chorus' (M)
Handel, 'Zadok the Priest' (E)
George Harrison, 'My Sweet Lord' (P)
Haydn, *The Creation* (J)

Haydn, Symphony No. 101, 'The Clock' (M)
Roger Hodgson in Concert, Stuttgart 2013 (P)
Rupert Holmes, 'Escape' ('The Pina Colada Song') (J)
Hummel, Piano Concerto in B Minor (Stephen Hough) (N)

The Isley Brothers, 'This Old Heart of Mine' (K)

Karl Jenkins, 'Benedictus' (E)

Chaka Khan, 'Sleep On It' (S)

Lighthouse Family, 'High' (L)
Lighthouse Family, 'Ocean Drive' (L)
The Lord's Prayer, private recording sung by a friend (T)
Raul Lovisoni and Francesco Messina, *Prati Bagnati Del Monte Analogo* (S)

Madonna, 'Hung Up' (A)
Alanis Morissette, 'Thank You' (K)
Mozart, Cassation in B Flat Major, K 99, Menuet (L)
Mozart, Clarinet Concerto (C)
Mozart, Clarinet Quintet (J)
Mozart, *Cosí Fan Tutte* (P)
Mozart, *Requiem* (M)
Sarah McLachlan, 'Blackbird' (L)
Mahler, Symphony No. 2, 'The Resurrection' (Janet Baker) (S)
Mahler, 'Lieder eines fahrenden Gesellen' (J)
Mahler, 'Ich bin der Welt abhanden gekommen' (Janet Baker and John Barbirolli) (N)
Mahler, Symphony No. 5, Adagietto (C)
Mahler, Symphony No. 5 (Leonard Bernstein) (JF)
Myfanwy (both Welsh songs) (P)
Ennio Morricone, 'Gabriel's Oboe' (P)
Johnny Mathis and Neil Diamond, 'Love is Everything' (C)
Monteverdi, *Orfeo* (V)
Chris Montez, 'Let's Dance' (R)

Only Boys Aloud, 'Calon Lân' (N)
Only Boys Aloud, 'Gwahoddiad' (N)
Beccy Owen, 'Lullaby' (V)

Arvo Pärt, 'Passio' (C)
Dolly Parton, *Here You Come Again* (F)
Pergolesi, *Stabat Mater* (Nathalie Stutzmann and Philippe Jaroussky) (I)
Purcell, 'An Evening Hymn' (L)
Les Poules à Colin, 'La Fleur du Bois' (O)
Prokofiev, *Peter and the Wolf* (narrated by Wilfred Pickles) (H)

Queen, 'The Show Must Go On' (A)
Queen, 'Don't Stop Me Now' (P)

Rachmaninov, 'Rhapsody on a Theme of Paganini' (S)
Joshua Radin and Sheryl Crow, 'Beautiful Day' (L)
Renegade Soul, 'Everybody's Free' (L)

Schubert, Fantasie in F Minor for Four Hands (Radu Lupu and Murray Perahia)
    (H)
Schubert, Piano Quintet in A Major, 'The Trout' (H and P)
Schubert, Sonata in B Flat, D 960 (J)
Schubert, String Quartet in C Major (M)
Schubert, Symphony No. 5, first movement (M)
Schubert, 'An Die Musik' (R)
Shostakovich, String Quartets (P)
Sibelius, 'Intermezzo' from the Karelia Suite (J)
Simon and Garfunkel, 'Bridge Over Troubled Water' (I and S)
Sousa, 'The Liberty Bell' march (J)
Bruce Springsteen, 'Dancing in the Dark' ((P)
Bruce Springsteen, 'Thunder Road' (S)
Stanford, 'The Blue Bird' (D and J)
Cat Stevens, 'Morning Has Broken' (A)
'Suo Gân' (P)
Nina Simone, 'I Wish I Knew How It Would Feel To Be Free' (H and P)
John Sheppard, 'Libera Nos, Salva Nos' (M)
Richard Strauss, Four Last Songs (D)
Richard Strauss, Der Rosenkavalier, final trio (F)
The Shins, 'Saint Simon' (M)
Labi Siffre, 'Something Inside So Strong' (C)

Jake Thackray, 'The Blacksmith and the Toffeemaker' (S)
Tchaikovsky, Violin Concertos (C)
Jethro Tull, 'Bourée' (A)
Charles Trenet, 'La Mer' (C)
Tallis, 'Spem in Alium' (J)
Tallis, 'If Ye Love Me' (Rutter's arrangement) (S)

Van Morrison, 'Cypress Avenue' (L)
Vaughan Williams, 'Fantasia on a Theme by Thomas Tallis' (E)
Vaughan Williams, 'The Lark Ascending' (A)
Verdi, La Traviata (C)
Victoria, 'O Vos Omnes' (not 'Tenebrae') (S)

Westlake, Compassion (N)
Pharrell Williams, 'Happy' (A)
Jackie Wilson, '(Your Love Keeps Lifting Me) Higher and Higher' (K)
Bill Withers, 'Lovely Day' (L)
Bill Withers, 'Lean on Me' (S)

Acknowledgements

The Dear Readers remain anonymous to all except me. There are good reasons for this and I will name you only in my mind now, as I write to acknowledge you. You give me your close attention, and you lovingly accompany every step of my journey. I would not be who I am, this book would not be what it is, without you. Together we demonstrate the fundamentally social nature of human beings and the healing effect of loving porosity. Thank you.

My family feels like my own self at its most stalwart, challenging me to be strong and steady throughout the long journey. Thank you Paul, John, Anne, Monica, Fiona, Graham, Ivan, Jack, Sheila and Lisa.

The warmth of my Irish cousins; the neighbourliness of Knockanure, of Jean-François, Carla and the nursery tots, Rohit and Aisha, Paul and Joyce in Borough; the steady wit of my Ealing friends; the iconoclastic embrace of my Hastings friends; the depth of Eamonn; the unfailing, creative communications of Juliet, Barbara and Ian; the motets and bonhomie of St Michael's Chorale; and the generosity of Hyfield Stables have embraced me and supported me beyond anything I could have expected. My thanks to you all.

I am bound in gratitude to the clinical and support staff at Guy's and St Thomas and University College London Hospitals, you who achieve extraordinary levels of competence combined with humanity.

I am equally bound to my fellow myeloma patients who have walked the path before me and lit my way by their example, especially Donna and Francesca. I am grateful to all my fellow cancer patients in the chemotherapy village at Guy's, who keep on giving me strength by being different and interesting and human and enduring.

Westminster Abbey could never just be a place of employment. The professionalism and flair of my colleagues ensure that I can undergo treatment without fear of the work going awry, and also its pastoral wings and its beating, praying heart carry me. I especially want to thank you, Kathleen, Jane, Aneta, Mark, Paul, Lorraine, Jamie, Anthony, the Institute's Council of Reference and all its Fellows.

If the Dear Readers hadn't demonstrated it already, the team at Hodder would have shown me just how much a book is the fruit of many people's work. Katherine Venn, editor, you understood the script and encouraged me with your poetic response to its words. Rachael Duncan has been brilliant at publicity. Jessica Lacey's patience and Anne-Marie Greatorex's attention to the detail of copy-editing have been exemplary. My thanks are for you all.

Ruth Cairns, agent and friend, believed in the book and in me as an author. I cannot thank you enough for your skill, energy, laughter and integrity.

Laura Wilson knows me and knows good writing inside out. You gave me the courage I needed to publish and I will always be grateful.

My gratitude to Seán is too deep for words.

Notes

Prologue

1 François Mitterand, Prologue, in Marie de Hennezel, *Intimate Death: How the Dying Teach Us to Live*, trans Carol Brown Janeway (New York: Warner Books, 1995), p.ix.

I *Diagnosis*

1 Abigail Appleton, reproduced here with permission.
2 Anonymous saying.
3 Tristan Stone, reproduced here with permission.
4 Carol Bialock, 'Breathing Underwater' in *Coral Castles* (Fernwood Press, 2019), pp. 14-15. Used with permission.

II *First Part of the Treatment*

1 Gerard Manley Hopkins, 'Pied Beauty', in *Poems and Prose* (London: Penguin, 2008).
2 George Herbert, 'The Temper (I)', in *The Complete English Works*, ed. Ann Pasternak Slater (London: Random House, 1995).
3 'Lily the Pink', John Gormon, Mike McGear and Roger McGough, 1968.
4 George Herbert, 'The Temper (I)', in *Complete English Works*.
5 Gerard Manley Hopkins, 'My Own Heart', in *Poems and Prose*.
6 ibid.
7 Gerard Manley Hopkins, 'No Worst', in *Poems and Prose*.
8 Ted Hughes, 'The Horses', in *Collected Poems of Ted Hughes*, ed. Paul Keegan (London: Faber, 2005). Used with permission.
9 Bernhard Schlink, *Self's Punishment*, trans Rebecca Morrison (London: Orion Books, 2005).
10 John Barton, *A History of the Bible: The Book and its Faiths* (London: Penguin, 2019).
11 And wrote about in my doctoral thesis: *Restoring Porosity and the Ecological Crisis: A Post-Ricoeurian Reading of the Julian of Norwich Texts* (King's College

London, 2018) accessible here: https://kclpure.kcl.ac.uk/portal/files/94606632/2018_Foster_Gilbert_Claire_1352686_ethesis.pdf.

12 George Herbert, 'The Call', in *Complete English Works*.

13 Stephanie Shirley, *Let It Go: My Extraordinary Story* (London: Penguin, 2019).

14 Claire Tomalin, *A Life of My Own* (London: Penguin, 2018).

15 Jared Diamond, 'Guide to Reducing Life's Risks', in the *New York Times*, 2013. https://www.nytimes.com/2013/01/29/science/jared-diamonds-guide-to-reducing-lifes-risks.html.

16 For more details of external evidence see my thesis, *Restoring Porosity*, Chapter 2.

17 Benedicta Ward, 'Julian the Solitary', in *Julian Reconsidered* (Oxford: SLG Press, 1995), pp. 11–29.

18 Peter Reason, *In Search of Grace: An Ecological Pilgrimage* (Alresford: John Hunt, 2017).

19 Philip Larkin, 'The Trees', in *The Complete Poems of Philip Larkin* (London: Faber, 2012).

20 George Herbert, 'Easter Wings', in *Complete English Works*.

21 *I'm Sorry I Haven't a Clue*, BBC Radio 4, https://www.bbc.co.uk/programmes/b006qnwb/episodes/guide.

22 Mary Colwell, *Curlew Moon* (London: HarperCollins, 2018); Helen Macdonald, *H is for Hawk* (London: Jonathan Cape, 2014).

23 Elizabeth Jennings, 'The Idler', in *The Collected Poems* (Oxford: Carcanet Press, 2012).

III *Second Part of the Treatment*

1 J's friend, Stephen Hancock, 'Keeping the Faith', reproduced here with permission.

2 Kate Gross, *Late Fragments: Everything I Want to Tell You about This Magnificent Life* (London: William Collins, 2015).

3 Martha Nussbaum, in an interview with Bill Moyers, 29 September 2011, https://www.youtube.com/watch?v=tWfK1E4L--c&list=PL-zebpgZ8d8Rju H7Ul13ujOoXY-V1aKlA&index=2.

4 Jocelyn Playfair, *A House in the Country* (London: Persephone Books, 2010 [1944]). Used with permission from persephonebooks.co.uk.

IV *Third Part of the Treatment*

1 Shelly von Strunckel, *Sunday Times*, 13 October 2019. For more information about astrology: www.shelleyvonstrunckel.com

2 D.H. Lawrence, 'Self-pity', in *Selected Poems*, ed. James Fenton (London: Penguin, 2008).

3 Helen Mosby, reproduced here with permission.

4 Alasdair Maclean, 'Fiona with a Fieldmouse', in *From The Wilderness* (London: Victor Gollancz, 1973).

5 George Gordon Byron, *Don Juan* (London: Penguin Classics, 2004), Canto II.

6 John Williams, *Augustus* (London: Vintage Classics, 2003).

7 John Williams, *Stoner* (London: Vintage Classics, 2012).
8 Tirzah Garwood, *Long Live Great Bardfield* (London: Persephone Books, 2016 [1935]).
9 Byron, *Don Juan*. Thank you again, J.
10 John Berger, *Bento's Sketchbook* (London: Verso, 2011), p. 72.
11 Charles Dickens, *Barnaby Rudge* (London: The Folio Society, 1987 [1841]), p. 582.
12 David Omand, *Securing the State* (London: Hurst Publishers, 2011).

V *Maintenance Chemotherapy and Covid-19*

1 Edward Carpenter, 'The Lake of Beauty' in *Towards Democracy* (London: Routledge, 2017 [1888]).
2 Alexander of Hales, Alexandri Alensis, *Angli Summae Theologiae*: Pars Quarta (hereafter, SH Bk IV),Q26, M3, Ar7 (Cologne: Sumptibus Ioannis Gymnici, sub Monocerote, 1622), p 721: 'Legitur enim de B. Greg. quod cum purgarert ve[n]trem, et Psalmum diceret, apparuit ei diabolus, quaerens quid faceret; et respondit: "ventrem meum purgo, et Deum meum laudo; opera enim natura perfectis turpia non videntur".'
3 *Spitting Image*, created by Roger Law and archived at Cambridge University.
4 Fra Giovanni Giocondo (c. 1435–1515), prayer from his letter to Countess Allagia Aldobrandeschi, Christmas Eve, 1513.
5 Mary Oliver, *Upstream: Selected Essays* (New York: Penguin, 2016), pp. 18–19.
6 Bryan Robertson, director of the Whitechapel Art Gallery from 1957, on what he looked for in art.
7 Collect for Ash Wednesday, *Book of Common Prayer*.
8 Unknown source.
9 The prisoners' dilemma was devised by Flood and Dresher in 1950 and poses the following: two prisoners, A and B, interrogated separately, are both offered choices between testifying against the other or remaining silent. If A testifies against B and B remains silent, A will be let off and B will receive ten years' imprisonment, and *vice versa*. If both A and B testify against each other, both will receive two years' imprisonment. If both remain silent, both will receive six months' imprisonment, the maximum sentence the court can give in the absence of evidence.